WALKING BOSTON

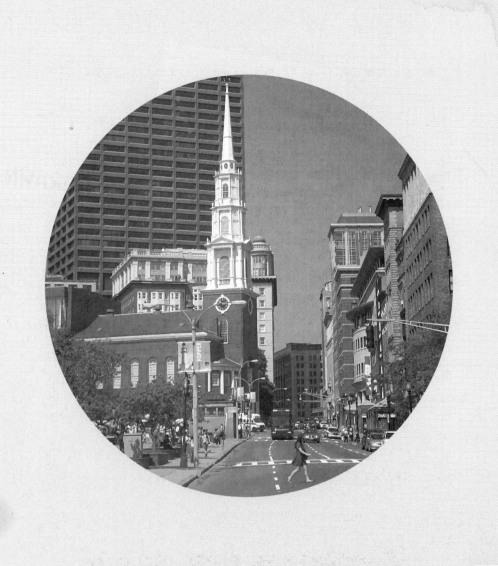

WALKING BOSTON

34 tours through
Beantown's cobblestone streets,
historic districts, ivory towers,
and new waterfront

Robert Todd Felton

WILDERNESS PRESS · BERKELEY, CA

Walking Boston: 34 tours through Beantown's cobblestone streets, historic districts,
       ivory towers, and new waterfront

1st EDITION July 2008

Copyright © 2008 by Robert Todd Felton

Front cover photos copyright © 2008 by Robert Todd Felton
Interior photos by Robert Todd Felton, except for the following: Hillary Pember, pp. 9, 49, 69, 85,
  89, 189, 195, and 219; Betsy Archer, p. 236
Maps: Bart Wright, Lohnes + Wright
Cover and book design: Larry B. Van Dyke and Lisa Pletka
Book layout: Beverly Butterfield, Girl of the West Productions
Book editor: Eva Dienel

ISBN 978-0-89997-448-4
UPC 7-19609-97448-2

Manufactured in Canada

Published by: Wilderness Press
                1345 8th Street
                Berkeley, CA 94710
                (800) 443-7227; FAX (510) 558-1696
                info@wildernesspress.com
                www.wildernesspress.com

Visit our website for a complete listing of our books and for ordering information.

Cover photos: (*Front, clockwise from bottom center*) Financial District, Faneuil Hall, Public Garden, Christopher
              Columbus Park, swan boats in the Public Garden, Harvard, and the Charles River;
              (*Back, clockwise from bottom left*) Copley Square Farmer's Market, Custom House Tower, and
              shade pavilion on Spectacle Island

Frontispiece: Park Street Church

SAFETY NOTICE: Although Wilderness Press and the author have made every attempt to ensure that the information in this book is accurate at press time, they are not responsible for any loss, damage, injury, or inconvenience that may occur to anyone while using this book. You are responsible for your own safety and health while following the walking trips described here. Always check local conditions, know your own limitations, and consult a map.

To my mother and grandmother,
whose Quincy roots gave this project special resonance

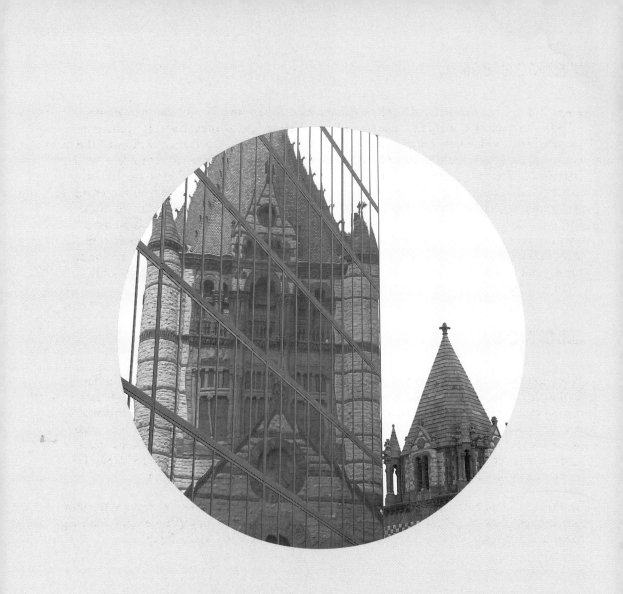

Trinity Church reflected in the John Hancock Tower

acknowledgments

Every book needs friends, and I am very thankful for the many friends who stepped up to help this project along. First, thanks to Laura Keresty and Roslyn Bullas for getting me involved with Wilderness Press. Eva Dienel at Wilderness Press was patient and insightful in her editing suggestions, and Laura Shauger stepped in ably to see the project to completion. Bart Wright created lovely maps, and Beverly Butterfield did a great job with the layout. Ethan Gilsdorf, Baer Tierkel, and Deborah Fraize were wonderfully gracious in suggesting walks and attractions. Jennifer Gilbert deserves special thanks for her contribution of the MIT walk as well as the Belle Isle and East Boston walks. Zaim Elkalai and his mother, Kathleen Traphagen, created the Jamaica Plain walk. Hillary Pember was a complete gift, fact-checking and hunting down the final details. And no journey, whether on paper or on the ground, would be complete without my own guides—my wife, Chris, and my sons, Liam and Tim.

author's note

When the first European settlers came to Boston, it was not much more than a collection of three rises at the end of a long, thin neck of land. As Boston grew by shearing off the tops of those hills and filling the bays, new neighborhoods were created and street patterns were irrevocably jumbled. So it is not surprising that there are few straight streets or grids in Boston (Back Bay is an exception). And with often poorly marked or ambiguous street signs, it may seem impossible to navigate Boston. The good news is that you are rarely far from a major landmark or historical district, so you are never hopelessly lost.

The walks in this book are designed to give the reader a sense of traveling through Boston's rich cultural heritage. Many of the walks can also be linked into longer routes, but don't try too much in a single outing. There is a lot to see and do on each walk. Enjoy!

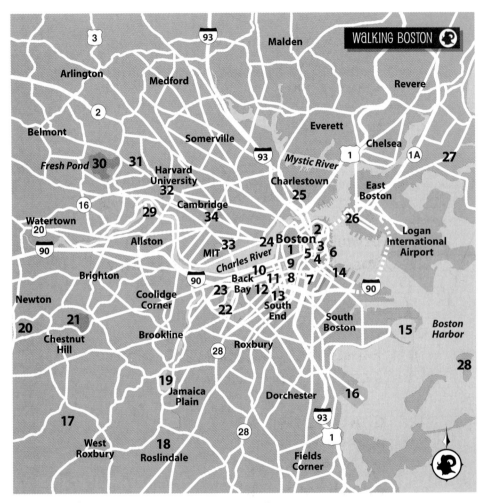

Numbers on this locator map correspond to Walk numbers.

TaBLe OF CONTeNTS

INTRODUCTION

Boston is a walker's town. It's as clear as the brick red path marking the Freedom Trail, the bright blue signs of the Harborwalk, and the green of the Emerald Necklace series of parks. Boston's nearly 400-year history has led to the development of hidden neighborhoods, historic sites, and iconic parks that tempt both Bostonians and visitors out onto the sidewalks, paths, and trails lacing this close-knit city. In addition, the Big Dig project, which helped revive downtown and the waterfront by moving Interstate 93 underground, has created an energy and excitement that has driven projects like the Harborwalk and the Rose Fitzgerald Kennedy Greenway. Neighborhoods like South Boston and the Bulfinch Triangle are experiencing new growth and positive development—and even established cultural attractions like the Children's Museum and the Boston Tea Party Museum are getting major facelifts. Not only are there now more opportunities for walking, there are sparkling new parks, cafes, and stores along old strolling avenues like Newbury St.

This makes it an exciting time to walk in Boston. The aim of this book is to offer you, the walker, the best of Boston's new and old rambles. Each walk is meant to be a complete experience in itself, so I've paired a legendary baseball stadium with a wonderful little Thai restaurant around the corner. You can view Boston's newest and most striking museum, and then get a lobster roll from a delightful wooden shack on Fort Point Channel.

A final caveat—although I tried to make each walk a complete experience, I did not cover Boston completely. Because Boston is so tightly packed with treasures around every corner, please forgive me if I overlooked your favorite spot or new discovery. And feel free to send me news and updates from your own rambles.

So, go ahead, lace up those shoes and take a walk. Whether you follow a red line, a blue sign, or the Emerald Necklace, you are always on the road to something special.

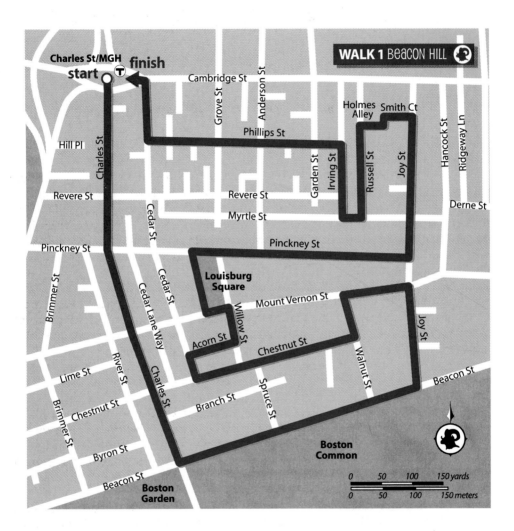

WALK 1 BeaCON HILL

Charles St/MGH — finish — start

Cambridge St

Anderson St

Grove St

Holmes Alley — Smith Ct

Phillips St

Hill Pl

Charles St

Garden St

Irving St

Russell St

Joy St

Hancock St

Ridgeway Ln

Revere St

Revere St

Derne St

Cedar St

Myrtle St

Pinckney St

Pinckney St

Brimmer St

Cedar St

Louisburg Square

Mount Vernon St

Joy St

Cedar Lane Way

Willow St

Acorn St

Chestnut St

Walnut St

River St

Lime St

Charles St

Branch St

Spruce St

Beacon St

Brimmer St

Chestnut St

Boston Common

Byron St

Beacon St

Boston Garden

0   50   100   150 yards
0   50   100   150 meters

1 BEACON HILL: COBBLESTONES AND GASLIGHTS

BOUNDARIES: Charles St., Beacon St., Joy St., Cambridge St.
DISTANCE: Approx. 2 miles
DIFFICULTY: Moderate
PARKING: Charles St. Parking Garage at 144 Charles St.; Boston Common Parking Garage on Charles St.
PUBLIC TRANSIT: Charles St./MGH T Station on the Red Line; busses 43 and 55

San Francisco has Nob Hill, Manhattan has Park Avenue, and London has Belgravia—neighborhoods where heritage, architecture, and money are inextricably linked. For Boston, it's Beacon Hill, a maze of cobblestone streets and well-kept row houses arranged along Beacon Hill between Storrow Drive and the State House. The neighborhood is a National Historic District, an elite enclave of privilege, and a vibrant community—all in one. It's the type of place where you can live just down the street from both the Museum of African American History and Senator John Kerry.

Beacon Hill comes alive in early spring when window boxes and flowering pear trees explode into color. And if a passing thundershower forces you to duck into one of the many good cafes or shops along Charles St., so much the better. If you take this walk at dusk, you'll appreciate the gas lamps throughout Beacon Hill that still burn 24 hours a day. The lamps are just one of the many details, like brass door knockers and ornate ironwork, which give Beacon Hill its considerable charm.

● Begin at the Charles St./MGH T Station and head south on Charles St., toward the Boston Common. Charles St. is Beacon Hill's town square. Pass through here on any evening and enjoy the jostling camaraderie of residents picking up dinner or dry cleaning. The mix of stores is wonderfully eclectic, with trendy clothing boutiques and hardware shops standing cheek by jowl with important historical sites.

One of those sites was on the right, at 148 Charles St., the former site of the James T. Fields House, which was torn down and replaced with a parking garage in the early 20th century. It's a shame to think that cars are now parked on the site where Fields, the renowned 19th-century publisher, gathered many of America's foremost thinkers and writers, like Nathaniel Hawthorne, Ralph Waldo Emerson, and Henry Wadsworth Longfellow, for dinner parties at his house.

Walk down Charles St. to the Charles Street Meeting House, on the right, at 70 Charles St. (the corner of Charles and Mt. Vernon St.). Built in 1804, this former white Baptist church became the African Methodist Episcopal Church in 1876 and echoed with the voices of important abolitionists like William Lloyd Garrison, Harriet Tubman, and Frederick Douglass. In 1920, the church was saved from the wrecking ball by being relocated 10 feet toward the river to make room for an expanded Charles St. Note the cupola that is in place of the traditional steeple often used for New England churches; it seemed to foreshadow its current, more secular use as a cafe and stores.

Continue on Charles St. If you're in the mood to stop, try one of the sandwiches on freshly baked baguettes or a great salad from Cafe Bella Vita, on the right at 30 Charles St. Alternatively, you can a grab a few groceries and a good bottle of wine for a picnic from DeLuca's Market, on the left at 11 Charles St. These cafes and markets, along with their quaint store signs and the cobblestone street, give Charles St. a European feel. Walking past DeLuca's brings you to the corner of Charles and Beacon streets (there's a Starbucks here). From here, you can see the Boston Common stretching out to the left and up the hill, and the Public Garden on the left side of Charles St.

- Turn left at the corner with the Starbucks and head up the hill on Beacon St. Facing the Common are the former homes of judges, ministers, and public figures.

- Turn left on Joy St. and walk to 5 Joy St., home of the Appalachian Mountain Club (open weekdays only). Located in a little brick house, this recreation and advocacy group for the Northeast offers a variety of programs and suggestions for those looking to leave the city behind. Its bookstore is stocked with great guides and maps for the New England area. You do not need to be a member of the club to use the resources.

- Turn left on Mt. Vernon St. and walk just down the hill to 55 Mt. Vernon, the Nichols House Museum, which was once the home of activist and philanthropist Rose Standish Nichols, who stipulated in her will that her 1804 Charles Bulfinch-designed house and eclectic collection of Victorian and Colonial furniture be open to the public. Take the $5 tour to see the Bulfinch architectural details and dark Victorian furnishings, but more importantly to learn about this fascinating and bold woman. She was a suffragette, author, and landscape designer in an age when women were supposed to keep house and gardens, not design them.

- Continue downhill, and, as you walk, note the carefully preserved elm trees that lend the street so much of its leafy serenity. Other notable details include the wide variety of brass door knockers, boot scrapers, and ironwork.

- Turn left on Walnut St.

- Make a quick right on Chestnut St. to continue down the hill. The houses at 13, 15, and 17 Chestnut are perhaps the nicest wedding presents one can give. Wealthy Boston merchant James Swan and his wife, Hepzibah, gave one to each daughter in the early 19th century on the occasion of their nuptials. Designed by Charles Bulfinch, the houses have marble columns and recessed arches.

- Continue down the street to 29A Chestnut and note the windows of the house of actor Edwin Booth (brother of John Wilkes Booth, who assassinated President Abraham Lincoln). Their purple tint is the result of a manufacturing defect that caused the glass to turn purple when exposed to air. Although it happened accidentally, these windows were viewed as prettier than normal windows and quickly became a must-have fashion in Victorian Boston. Keep your eye out for them throughout Beacon Hill.

Acorn Street

BaCK STOrY: CHarLeS BULFINCH

Born in Boston in 1763, Charles Bulfinch attended Harvard before settling into his career as America's first native-born professional architect. He established his practice by designing many of the houses on Beacon Hill before being tapped to design the Massachusetts State House, which was begun on July 4, 1797.

After that, he went on to enlarge Faneuil Hall, design numerous churches, like St. Stephen's Catholic Church in the North End, and design private homes, including three for Harrison Gray Otis, a prominent Boston politician and developer of Beacon Hill. Known for his intelligent use of brick and granite and the stately elegance of his public buildings, Bulfinch is credited with transforming much of Boston from a wooden port town to an impressive 19th-century metropolis. However, Bulfinch was better at design than financial management, and in 1811, his debts sent him to jail—ironically in a prison of his own design.

In 1818, President James Monroe offered Bulfinch $2,500 a year for 12 years to help design the U.S. Capitol. Although some of his details have been replaced, much of the Bulfinch-designed Capitol Building remains.

● Turn right on W. Cedar St. and follow it one block to Acorn St.

● Turn right on Acorn. This narrow alley has been called the most photographed street in the world. While that may be an exaggeration, the steep street, with its gaslights, grass growing between the cobblestones, and classic Victorian houses is certainly worth setting up your tripod.

● Turn left on Willow St. and follow it to Louisburg Square.

● Veer left across Mt. Vernon St. and then veer right to take the west (downhill side) of Louisburg Square. Louisa May Alcott, whose 19th-century novel *Little Women* is an American classic, lived her last days in the fine house at 10 Louisburg Square. Although her childhood included other residences on Beacon Hill (at 20, 43, and

81 Pinckney St.), the runaway success of *Little Women* allowed her to move into the more fashionable Louisburg Square toward the end of her life.

● Turn right on Pinckney St. for additional examples of Beacon Hill's literary pedigree. But first, a bit of its current glamour: At the northeast corner of Pinckney and Louisburg Square is the home of former presidential candidate and U.S. Senator John Kerry. But don't linger too long in front of the $7 million house; the Secret Service will take note.

Instead, climb the hill toward Joy St. American novelist Nathaniel Hawthorne, who wrote *The Scarlet Letter* and *Mosses from an Old Manse,* lived at 54 Pinckney, and a young Henry David Thoreau lived at 4 Pinckney well before his sojourn at Walden Pond.

● At the top of the hill, turn left on Joy St. After you crest the hill and descend toward Cambridge St., you come to the Museum of African American History, at 46 Joy St. The museum, which consists of the African Meeting House and the Abiel Smith School, honors and celebrates Boston's, and especially Beacon Hill's, role in advocating for the rights of slaves. The meeting house, built in 1806 primarily with black labor and funds from both the white and black communities, served as the focal point for the New England abolition movement. It was here that the white abolitionist William Lloyd Garrison founded the New England Anti-Slavery Society, which helped drive the campaign to abolish slavery as well as assist escaped slaves in finding freedom. It was also here that escaped slave and leader Frederick Douglass gave a speech after being run out of Tremont Temple. This is the oldest black church still standing in the United States and offers a wide variety of exhibits and programs exploring African-American history.

Next door, Abiel Smith School offers a sense of what life was like for African-American elementary students in the 1800s. Operating as a school from 1835 to 1855, this was the first building in the nation constructed as a public school for black children. The interior has been renovated and reconstructed with displays featuring examples of mid-19th-century education.

- Turn left to head down Smith Ct. (right next door to the museum). The houses are typical of the ones owned by free blacks in the 19th century, before many of them migrated to South Boston.

- At the end of Smith Ct., turn left on tiny, winding Holmes Alley, where escaped slaves could flee from bounty hunters by either blending into the crowds of free blacks who gathered there or slipping behind doors in the alley. Slip down the alley yourself to access South Russell St.

- Turn left on S. Russell St.

- Turn right on Myrtle St. and go one block to Irving St.

- Turn right on Irving.

- Turn left on Phillips St. Just past Garden St., on the right, is Vilna Shul, the oldest synagogue in Boston and home to the Boston Center for Jewish Heritage. Stop in to gaze at the stained glass Star of David and the sanctuary flooded with natural light from three skylights.

- Continue three blocks to the Lewis and Harriet Hayden House, at 66 Phillips St. Although the house is now private and you'll have to admire it from the outside, the front porch is actually the most interesting part. According to local legend, kegs of gunpowder were stored underneath the front porch so that when slave hunters came to this stop on the Underground Railroad, the Haydens (Lewis himself was an escaped slave) could greet the white men with lit candles and threaten to drop them on the gunpowder below the porch if they tried to come inside.

- After the Hayden House, turn right on W. Cedar St., which runs out to Cambridge St.

- Turn left on Cambridge St.

- Turn right on Charles St. to return to your starting point.

POINTS OF INTEREST

Charles Street Meeting House 70 Charles St., Boston, MA 02114

Cafe Bella Vita 30 Charles St., Boston, MA 02114, 617-720-4505

DeLuca's Market 11 Charles St., Boston, MA 02114, 617-227-2117
Appalachian Mountain Club 5 Joy St., Boston, MA 02114, 617-523-0636
Nichols House Museum 55 Mt. Vernon St., Boston, MA 02114, 617-227-6993
Museum of African American History 46 Joy St., Boston, MA 02114, 617-725-0022
Vilna Shul/Boston Center for Jewish Heritage 18 Phillips St., Boston, MA 02114, 617-523-2324

route summary

1. Begin at the Charles St./MGH T Station and head south on Charles St.
2. Turn left on Beacon St.
3. Turn left on Joy St.
4. Turn left on Mt. Vernon St.
5. Turn left on Walnut St.
6. Turn right on Chestnut St.
7. Turn right on W. Cedar St.
8. Turn right on Acorn St.
9. Turn left on Willow St.
10. Veer left to cross Mt. Vernon St., and then veer right to take the west (downhill) side of Louisburg Square.
11. Turn right on Pinckney St.
12. Turn left on Joy St.
13. Turn left on Smith Ct.
14. Bear left on Holmes Alley.
15. Turn left on S. Russell St.
16. Turn right on Myrtle St.
17. Turn right on Irving St.
18. Turn left on Phillips St.
19. Turn right on W. Cedar St.
20. Turn left on Cambridge St.
21. Turn right on Charles St. to return to your starting point.

Beacon Hill

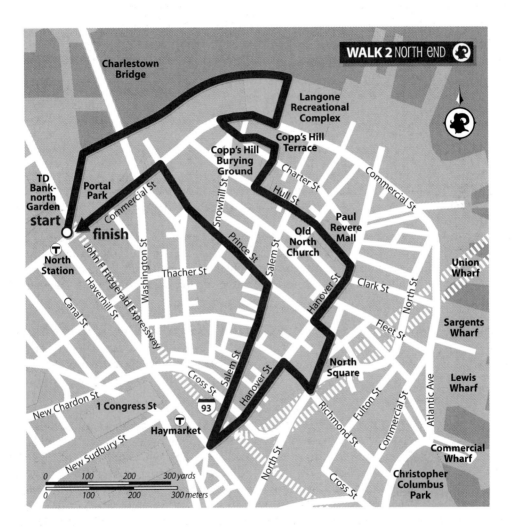

Charlestown Bridge

Langone Recreational Complex

Copp's Hill Terrace

Copp's Hill Burying Ground

Charter St

Hull St

Commercial St

TD Bank-north Garden

Portal Park

start

Commercial St

finish

Snowhill St

Paul Revere Mall

Old North Church

North Station

John F Fitzgerald Expressway

Washington St

Thacher St

Prince St

Salem St

Hanover St

Clark St

North St

Union Wharf

Haverhill St

Canal St

Fleet St

Sargents Wharf

Salem St

Cross St

Hanover St

North Square

Lewis Wharf

New Chardon St

1 Congress St

93

Fulton St

Commercial St

Atlantic Ave

Richmond St

Commercial Wharf

Haymarket

New Sudbury St

North St

Cross St

Christopher Columbus Park

0   100   200   300 yards
0   100   200   300 meters

10

2 NOrTH eND: ONe IF BY LaND, TWO FOr reaLLY GOOD Pasta IN BOSTON'S HISTOric aND DeLeCTaBLe DISTrICT

BOUNDARIES: Commercial St., Cross St., Atlantic Ave.
DISTANCE: Approx. 2 miles
DIFFICULTY: Moderate
PARKING: There are many paid parking lots in the area, but the Parcel 7 parking lot at 136 Blackstone St. offers discounts with North End restaurant validations.
PUBLIC TRANSIT: North Station T Station on the Orange and Green lines; busses 6, 92, 93, and 111

Boston's North End is all about the scents. Bakeries, pasta shops, cheese vendors, busy wharves, and bustling Italian restaurants all contribute their aromas. Merely wandering around the North End can make you hungry. And when the North End's fascinating history, from a clandestine Revolutionary War signal to a brilliant bank heist, is included, the result is one of Boston's finest walks.

Although the waterside parks and blooming flowers make spring and summer tempting, this is a great walk for wintertime. Cold weather cuts down on crowds, and, more importantly, gives you a good excuse to stop into one of the North End's famous Italian eateries. So, pack an appetite, get some good shoes (there's a lot of uneven pavement), and get going.

● Begin at the North Station T Station, which lies underneath the TD Banknorth Garden, at 100 Legends Way. The Banknorth Garden opened as the Fleet Center in 1995, and this concrete monster is home to both the Boston Celtics basketball team and the Boston Bruins hockey team. The building replaced the Boston Garden, which was modeled on Madison Square Garden and hosted its last game on September 6, 1995. For more stories and to see some athletic artifacts of the Celtics and Bruins dynasties, visit the Sports Museum of New England on the Banknorth Garden's fifth and sixth floors. The collection includes the penalty box from the old Boston Garden hockey rink, a piece of the parquet floor from the basketball court, and exhibits celebrating each of the Red Sox's World Series Championships.

- From the Banknorth Garden, head north-east on Causeway St., which becomes Commercial St. when it passes over Interstate 93. Stop at Portal Park on the left to gaze at the Leonard P. Zakim Bunker Hill Bridge. The park is just one of the many green spaces created downtown as a result of Boston's massive Big Dig construction project. The project, which included submerging Interstate 93 under the city and adding tunnels and bridges, cost nearly $15 billion and took more than 15 years to complete. The upside is that it greatly improved Boston's downtown and added a number of parks like Portal.

- Facing the Zakim Bridge, turn right and head for the Celtics cloverleaf painted on the side of the building. Take the stairs down to the Harborwalk, the paved path along the water (look for the blue signs with the white sailboat logo), and follow it north to the Langone Recreational Complex. This park was designed by Frederick Law Olmsted's firm in 1894 and has been renovated to include public bathrooms, bocce courts, tennis courts, and baseball/softball diamonds. In the winter, the Steriti Memorial Rink is open for public skating (call 617-523-9327 for hours and fees).

- After playing in the playground, turn right on Commercial St. and follow it to Charter St.

Back Story: The Big Brown Monster

It was more than 30 feet high and weighed 14,000 tons. It was a monster that left 21 people dead and more than 150 injured in its wake. It was 2.3 million gallons of molasses.

On January 15, 1919, a large steel tank near the corner of Foster and Commercial streets burst open, sending a huge wave of the dark, sticky syrup cascading down the streets of the North End. The company that owned the tank, U.S. Industrial Alcohol, which used the syrup in the production of alcohol, claimed that someone had sabotaged the tank. However, that theory was never proved, and the company was forced to pay out more than $1 million to the victims' families. In all, the disaster caused more than $100 million in property damage.

● Turn left on Charter. Walk up the hill to entrance of the Copp's Hill Burying Ground on the right. The gates are just past the Copp's Hill Terrace, a nice resting place on the left with a view out over the water. From Copp's Hill Terrace, you can also get a glimpse of Commercial St. (down and to the left), where Boston once experienced a serious and unexpected sugar high (see "Back Story: The Big Brown Monster").

● Exit Copp's Hill Terrace and cross Charter to enter the Copp's Hill Burying Ground. Copp's Hill is Boston's second oldest burial ground, and its gravestones date back to the mid-1600s. Make your way south along the path through the center of the grounds, and look for the graves of people like Increase and Cotton Mather—Colonial-era ministers famous for their anti-witchcraft rhetoric and literary accomplishments. Also check out the pockmarked gravestones (look for the grave of Daniel Malcon), which were used for target practice by the British soldiers who occupied Copp's Hill during the American Revolution.

● Exit the cemetery through the gates on the southern side, and turn left to walk east on Hull St. The Spite House, at 44 Hull, is a tiny building, only 10 feet wide and four stories high. According to local lore, the house was built in the 19th century to block the sunlight from a neighbor's house. Another story has it being built to block the view of the water. In any case, it's a private residence now, so you'll have to take your pictures from the outside.

● At the corner of Salem St., at 193 Salem, is one of the finest sanctuaries around, the Old North Church. This large brick and white clapboard structure is the oldest church building still standing in Boston. It still operates as an Episcopal church and is open to the public. Step inside to admire the immaculate space with the historic pews and furnishings.

North End

This church is also famous for its role in the American Revolution. According to the prearranged plan, Robert Newman, the church's sexton, quietly climbed the steps to the bell tower on the night of April 18, 1775, carrying two lanterns. If he had lit just the one lantern, it would have alerted fellow patriots across the river in Charlestown that British forces intended to march over Boston Neck, the spit of land that then connected Boston with the mainland. But he lit two lanterns, which signaled that the Redcoats were sailing up the Charles River before marching on Lexington and Concord. After the message went out, riders, including the now famous Paul Revere, set out to warn the people of Lexington and Concord of the approaching British Army. This ride (think: "The British are coming! The British are coming!") and the ensuing battles of Lexington and Concord pushed the colonies toward independence. Today, this time period is commemorated on the third Monday of each April as Patriot's Day, a state holiday that features Revolutionary War reenactments, a Red Sox day game at Fenway Park, and the running of the Boston Marathon.

● Follow the brick path between the church and the accompanying bookstore to the Paul Revere Mall (also called the "Prado" by the locals), behind the church. Although the mall has plaques and memorials to famous North Enders, the center is dominated by a Cyrus Dallin statue of Paul Revere atop his horse—so you can get a visual of what his ride might have looked like.

● Exit the Paul Revere Mall at Hanover St. On the opposite side of the street from the mall is St. Stephen's Church, at 401 Hanover St., another lovely and historical brick and white wood affair. Rose Kennedy (matriarch of the Kennedy clan) was baptized here in 1891. It is the last remaining church designed by Boston architect Charles Bulfinch.

● Turn right on Hanover St. and walk to Mike's Pastry, at 300 Hanover. Long a North End fixture, this Italian bakery attracts a steady stream of locals and visitors, who leave clutching the distinctive white and blue boxes. Step inside the warm, cheerful shop and listen to the banter between the clerks and regulars as you peruse the long glass cases filled with goodies. The famous cannoli are baked fresh, and the black and white cookies are soft and nearly a meal in themselves. You can't really go wrong, so make your choice and watch the staff deftly tie up the packages with string hanging from the ceiling.

- Turn left on Prince St. and walk one block to North Square.

- Turn right on North Square. Although it's chock full of historic buildings, a restaurant, and a postage-stamp sized park, the main attraction of the square is the Paul Revere House Museum, at 19 North Square. Here, you can investigate the life of this remarkable hero of the American Revolution. Born in 1734, Revere was a successful metalworker (he crafted silver tea services, church bells, and the copper roof of the Massachusetts State House on Beacon Street) before he became a well-known revolutionary rabble-rouser, who secretly rode through the countryside to warn the Minute Men of Lexington and Concord that the British Army was on the way.

  Next door to the Revere House is one of the oldest brick homes in the city. Built in 1710 for Moses Pierce, a Boston window-maker, the Pierce-Hichborn House was later owned by Nathaniel Hichborn, Paul Revere's cousin. Both houses are available for tours.

- Head to the south corner of North Square (like many "squares" in Boston, North Square is not a square at all but more of a triangle), and turn right on Richmond St.

- After one block, turn left on Hanover St. and walk one block. The distance is short, but it may take you a while. This section of Hanover is packed with great Italian eateries and cafes. In warmer weather, the streets are often crowded with old gentlemen smoking away the afternoons, hordes of tourists hunting down the perfect restaurant, and locals stopping to chat with their favorite merchants. In August, this street regularly fills with revelers during several festivals and feasts in honor of various patron saints. One of the most famous is the Feast of St. Anthony, on the last weekend of August. Get there early to follow the statue of St. Anthony as it is hoisted aloft and paraded through the North End.

- At the corner of Hanover and Cross St., you will see the North End Parks. Opened on November 5, 2007, these two parks (bisected by Hanover St.) provide a transition area from the more residential feel of the North End to the busier and more commercial downtown and Faneuil Hall districts. The designers call the parks North End's "front porch" and indeed, they are ideally situated for you to sit back, relax, and watch the world zip by—much like a good front porch.

- Cross Cross St. to enter the western parcel (on the right) and walk toward Blackstone St. Views of the Zakim Bridge and the Banknorth Garden open up to the west, and you can gaze down much of the Rose Fitzgerald Kennedy Greenway on the left.

- As you reach the end of the path, turn sharply right to head north again on the path leading toward Salem St. Note the patterned granite of the paths, the water features, the magnolias, ash, and flowering vines that reflect the cultural heritage of the area.

- Exit the park by crossing Cross St. and walking north on Salem St., one of the most calorie-laden avenues in all of Boston. Taste the toffee at Dairy Fresh Candies (57 Salem), sample a pizza slice from Antico Forno (93 Salem), peruse the pasta options at L'Osteria (104 Salem), or cap off a great meal with cappuccino and a cannoli at Bova Bakery (134 Salem). You won't—and shouldn't try to—go hungry here.

- If only to escape an imminent food coma, turn left on Prince St. and follow it three blocks to Commercial St. As you near Commercial, note the hulking parking garage just past the playground on the right, at 165 Prince. It was the site of what was the country's largest bank robbery in 1950, when seven masked men walked out of the Brink's Armored Car Company offices with close to $2.8 million in cash and securities. The case almost went unsolved (it was at the time the largest heist in America and called "the perfect crime") until one member confessed.

- At Commercial St., turn left and follow it to the North Station T Station. Note that Commercial becomes Causeway St. after Prince St.

POINTS OF INTEREST

TD Banknorth Garden 100 Legends Way, Boston, MA 02114, 617-624-1050

Langone Recreational Complex Commercial St. at Charter St., Boston, MA 02113, 617-626-1250

Copp's Hill Burying Ground Corner of Snowhill and Hull streets, Boston, MA 02113, 617-635-4505

Old North Church 193 Salem St., Boston, MA 02113, 617-523-6676

St. Stephen's Church 401 Hanover St., Boston, MA 02113, 617-523-1230

Mike's Pastry 300 Hanover St., Boston, MA 02113, 617-742-3050

Paul Revere House Museum/Pierce-Hichborn House 19 North Square, Boston, MA
02113, 617-523-2338

Dairy Fresh Candies 57 Salem St., Boston, MA 02113, 617-742-2639

Antico Forno 93 Salem St., Boston, MA 02113, 617-723-6733

L'Osteria 104 Salem St., Boston, MA 02113, 617-723-7847

Bova Bakery 134 Salem St., Boston, MA 02113, 617-523-5601

route summary

1.   Begin at the TD Banknorth Garden and head north on Causeway St. to Portal Park.

2.   Enter Portal Park and bear right on the path heading north toward the water.

3.   Exit Portal Park to the east and take the stairs down to Harborwalk.

4.   Follow the Harborwalk north to the North End Playground.

5.   Turn right on Commercial St.

6.   Turn left on Charter St.

7.   Turn right into Copp's Hill Burying Ground and walk south through the cemetery.

8.   Exit Copp's Hill Burying Ground on the south side and turn left on Hull St.

9.   At the corner of Hull and Salem streets, cut through the Old North Church square and
     the Paul Revere Mall to Hanover St.

10. Turn right on Hanover St.

11. Turn left on Prince St.

12. Turn right on North Square.

13. Turn right on Richmond St.

14. Turn left on Hanover St.

15. Cross over Cross St. to enter the North End Parks.

16. Follow the path west through the park until it stops.

17. Make a sharp right turn to follow the path north toward Salem St.

18. Exit the park at the junction of Cross and Salem streets and head north on Salem St.

19. Turn left on Prince St.

20. Turn left on Commercial St. (which becomes Causeway St.) and follow it to your starting point.

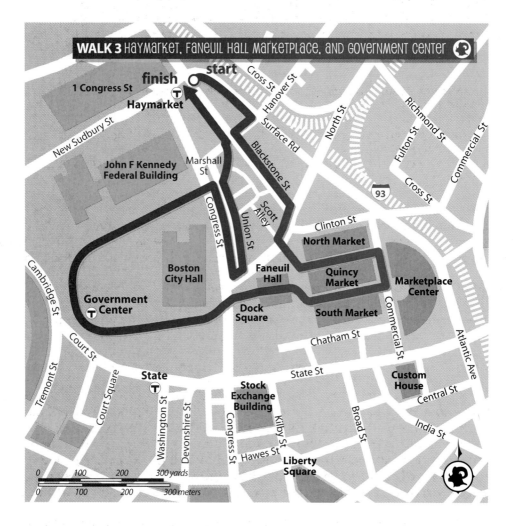

WALK 3 Haymarket, Faneuil Hall Marketplace, and Government Center

start

finish

1 Congress St

Ⓣ Haymarket

Cross St

Hanover St

New Sudbury St

John F Kennedy
Federal Building

Marshall
St

Surface Rd

North St

Richmond St

Fulton St

Commercial St

Blackstone St

93

Cross St

Congress St

Scott
Alley

Union St

Clinton St

North Market

Boston
City Hall

Faneuil
Hall

Quincy
Market

Marketplace
Center

Cambridge St

Government
Ⓣ Center

Dock
Square

South Market

Commercial St

Atlantic Ave

Court St

Chatham St

Tremont St

Court Square

State

Ⓣ

Washington St

Devonshire St

State St

Stock
Exchange
Building

Kilby St

Congress St

Broad St

Custom
House

Central St

India St

Hawes St

Liberty
Square

0   100   200   300 yards

0   100   200   300 meters

3 Haymarket, Faneuil Hall Marketplace, and Government Center: Marketing Boston

BOUNDARIES: **Surface Road, Chatham St., City Hall Plaza, New Chardon St.**
DISTANCE: **Approx. 1 mile**
DIFFICULTY: **Easy**
PARKING: **There are parking garages at 75 State St. and at Government Center Garage (50 New Sudbury St.).**
PUBLIC TRANSIT: **Haymarket T Station on the Green and Orange lines; busses 92, 93, 352, 353, and 354**

Located in the heart of Boston, the Faneuil Hall and Quincy Market areas are to Boston what Fisherman's Wharf and Pier 39 are to San Francisco: famous locales with historical significance reincarnated as tourist havens. This walk also visits Haymarket, one of the country's oldest and best farmer's markets, along with the basement meat shops along Blackstone St.

Although the time of year is not as important to this walk as the day of the week—Haymarket Farmer's Market is open rain, snow, or sunshine but only on Fridays and Saturdays—it's nice to do this walk in early summer, before the tourist hordes descend and just in time to see the flower market explode with color.

● **From the Haymarket T Station, follow Surface Rd. south to Hanover St.**

● **Veer right on Hanover and then veer left on Blackstone St. to continue south to North St. On Fridays and Saturdays, you may not make it far beyond the corner of Hanover and Blackstone, where the 200-year-old Haymarket Farmer's Market sets up shop. Well-known for both the volubility of the vendors and the discounts on the produce, Haymarket is a sight to see and hear. There is plenty of banter, shouting out of prices, some good-natured heckling, and lots of advertising from the 50 vendors (many of whom are carrying on a family tradition) arranged along this short block.**

If you miss the farmer's market, sneak down the stairs on the right-hand side to any one of the basement shops along Blackstone St. to check out the Halal meat

markets. Halal meats, like kosher foods, are processed and brought to market based on the strict requirements of Islamic law. Many of the city's African, Muslim, and Latino residents come to get their meats and cheeses here, and a visit to the belowground shops can be an intriguing introduction to these cultures.

- Turn right on North St. and walk a half block to Scott Alley, on the right. Cross to the south side of North St. and enter Faneuil Hall Marketplace in between the North Market and the Flower Market. The entire Faneuil Hall Marketplace consists of Faneuil Hall, the North and South markets, the Flower Market, and, most famously, Quincy Market. The three 535-foot-long and 50-foot-wide granite buildings that comprise North, South, and Quincy markets were the dream of Mayor Josiah Quincy. However, not everybody bought into the idea; it was dubbed "Quincy's Folly" during construction because many critics considered it an outlandish waste of time and money. Nonetheless, Quincy's steadfast determination to get the project done outlasted his opponents, and the markets opened in 1826.

- The easiest way to navigate Faneuil Hall Marketplace is simply to walk from one end to the other (from west to east), so turn left to wander down the alleyway between North Market and Quincy Market. North Market is filled with shops like Orvis, the Bill Rodgers Running Center, and Celtic Weavers. On the right are just some of the more than 40 pushcarts hawking everything from embroidered Boston Red Sox hats to batik prints. For a classic Beantown sit-down restaurant, try venerable Durgin-Park in the North Market building. The motto of the restaurant, which opened in 1826, is "established before you were born." In addition to its longevity, the restaurant is known for the quick wit and good-natured chiding of its waitstaff.

- From the easternmost end, turn right to enter the main hall of Quincy Market, where you'll find dozens of food counters offering everything from New England clam chowder to sushi. At the halfway point, stop to look up at the impressive dome over the central rotunda.

- Exit from the western side of Quincy Market, and continue straight across the plaza to cross through Faneuil Hall. (Don't neglect the bottom-floor markets in Faneuil Hall itself). Faneuil Hall was built in 1742 by Peter Faneuil (pronounced "Fan-yool"), a successful merchant who wanted to give the fledgling city a building for civic meetings.

The building was then enlarged by architect Charles Bulfinch in 1805. Although the ground floor is filled with shops and vendors, the upper floors continue to host public meetings, just as they have since Faneuil's day.

- Exit through the western side of Faneuil Hall and stop to take a look at the statue of Samuel Adams out front. Before he was revived as a brewer of beer (he actually had little to do with today's Samuel Adams beer brand—apparently he was a lousy beer-maker and businessman), Adams was a colonial merchant with fiery rhetoric and a willingness to take up arms against the British. His statue is in the middle of Dock Square, so named because it marks what in 1630 was the shoreline of Boston. This area is popular with buskers juggling flaming bowling pins or break dancing. There are more than 50 street performers with acts from around the world registered to perform in the Faneuil Hall Marketplace area.

- From Dock Square, cross to the western side of Congress St. and look for the stairs to the left of City Hall. Turn around to look up to see the 39-pound grasshopper weathervane on top of Faneuil Hall. It has fallen off in an earthquake and been stolen by ambitious thieves, but it now rests safely on the rooftop.

- Climb the stairs to Government Center Plaza to find City Hall, the John F. Kennedy Federal Office Building, and a lot of concrete. Called Scollay Square in its 1930s and '40s heyday, this site was home to racy burlesque shows and, oddly, the workshops of Alexander Graham Bell and Thomas Edison (you can see the plaque commemorating the first phone call in front of the J.F.K. Building on the western side).

Faneuil Hall

In an effort to clean up the area, which had become a prime destination for sailors on leave, young male students from the area's schools, and visiting business men, Scollay Square was torn down in the early 1960s. Interestingly, the two inventors are memorialized in the square's government buildings, but renowned Scollay Square performers like Rose la Rose—whose, um, "talents" brought thousands of visitors to Scollay Square—are not.

● Walk toward the southwest corner of the square, at the intersection of Government Center Plaza and Court St., and look for the bright copper teakettle over what is now a Starbucks. The kettle was first hung in 1875 outside the shop of the Oriental Tea Company, which held a contest to see who could guess how many gallons the kettle could hold. Thirteen people correctly guessed 227 gallons, 2 quarts, 1 pint, and three gills, and they shared the 40 pounds of tea offered as a prize. The kettle has been moved from location to location over the years, but now it hangs not far from its original spot, where it is fed steam from the furnaces of nearby buildings.

● From the teakettle, head north across the square to the J.F.K. Building, the monolith just past City Hall. If you find the bunker-like appearance of Boston's City Hall a bit disconcerting, you'll be relieved to learn that architectural historians call this particular building style "Brutalism." It may look like it was built of Legos, but the squat, grey, concrete structure is designed to give the illusion of permanence and importance. (It certainly doesn't look like it's going anywhere anytime soon.) Hurry down the stairs between City Hall and the J.F.K. Building to the western side of Congress St.

● Cross to the east side of Congress St. to the Holocaust Memorial. Dedicated in 1995, the Holocaust Memorial is a powerful reminder of the six Nazi death camps. Six 54-foot, steel-and-glass towers, inscribed with 6 million numbers representing those who died in the camps, are lined along a black granite path. Directly underneath each tower is a black grate inscribed with the name of one of the death camps. Steam rises from each of the grates, creating a chilling effect. Quotes from survivors and liberators are carved into the granite walls lining the path through the towers.

● Walk south along the path, under the towers, and continue straight to the James Michael Curley Park. The park's namesake, James Michael Curley, was one of

Boston's most beloved and controversial mayors. Known for his oratorical bluster and occasional run-ins with the law, he was elected for his third mayoral term in 1946, despite being indicted and later sentenced to jail for mail fraud. He's been memorialized in books and in the Mighty Mighty Bosstones' song "The Rascal King." You can come face to face with him with two statues at the southern end of the park.

● From the statues of Curley, cross to the east side of Union St. at the crosswalks, and turn left on Union to walk north. If you are feeling hungry, duck into Boston's most famous oyster joint, the Union Oyster House (at 41 Union), the oldest continually operating restaurant in the United States. The wait for a table can be long (and your reward is mediocre and overpriced prepared food), so try to get a seat at the long wooden bar and banter with the shuckers as they prepare a dozen fresh oysters for you to slurp down. Order the Daniel Webster dinner (six plates of oysters with six glasses of brandy), named for a famous Massachusetts statesman and lawyer in the 19th century. Another famous name associated with this place is Louis Philippe, the last king of France; he taught French in a boarding room above what is now the Oyster House.

● Continue down Union for just a few more doors to tiny Marshall St., which is actually more of an alleyway, and bear right. Walk one block to the Boston Stone Souvenir Shop. Face the front door and take a close look at the bottom of the wall on the right-hand side. There, almost hidden, is the Boston Stone. Originally used as a grindstone in the 17th century, it was placed in this wall in 1737. Many claim that it marked the geographic center of Boston and was used to calculate distances to Boston from outlying cities. While that has not been verified, it now serves as more of an oddity in this age of GPS technology.

● Walk another 20 steps on Marshall to reach Hanover St. and the familiar din of Haymarket. Turn right on Hanover and go one block to Surface Rd.

● Turn left on Surface Rd. to return to your starting point at the Haymarket T Station.

POINTS OF INTEREST

Haymarket Farmer's Market Corner of Blackstone and Hanover streets, Boston, MA 02109
Boston Halal Meat Market 114 Blackstone St., Boston, MA 02109, 617-367-6181
Faneuil Hall Marketplace Clinton St. and North St., Boston, MA 02109, 617-523-1300
Durgin-Park North Market, Boston, MA 02109, 617-227-2038
Union Oyster House 41 Union St., Boston, MA 02108, 617-227-2750
Boston Stone Souvenir Shop 9 Marshall St., Boston, MA 02108, 617-227-6968

route summary

1. From the Haymarket T Station, follow Surface Rd. south.

2. Veer right on Hanover St., and then make an immediate left on Blackstone St., heading south.

3. Turn right on North St. and walk to Scott Alley.

4. Enter Faneuil Hall Marketplace in between the North Market and the Flower Market.

5. Explore Faneuil Hall Marketplace by walking from west to east, and then return from east to west through Quincy Market.

6. Exit Faneuil Hall Marketplace at the western edge and cross to the west side of Congress St.

7. Ascend the stairs to the left of City Hall and walk to the southwest corner of Government Center Plaza, at Court St.

8. Head north across the square and descend the stairs between the J.F.K. Building and City Hall.

9. At the bottom of the stairs, cross to the east side of Congress St. to Holocaust Memorial Park.

10. Walk south through the park and exit by turning left to walk north on Union St.

11. Bear right on Marshall St.

12. Turn right on Hanover St.

13. Turn left on Surface Rd. to return to the Haymarket T Station.

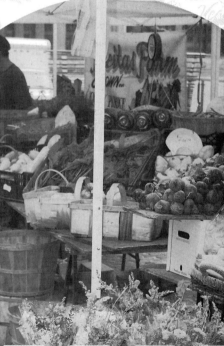

Government Center Farmer's Market

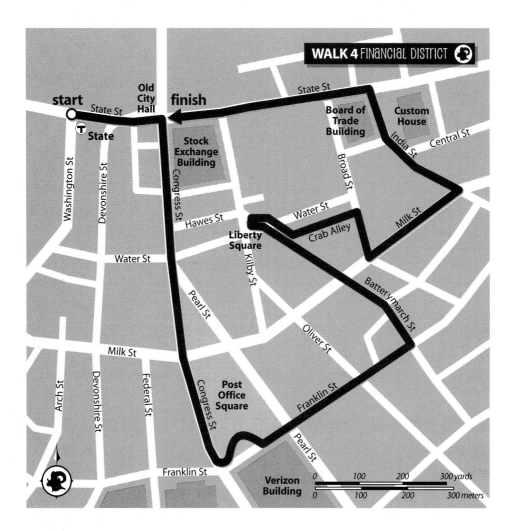

start

State

State St

Old City Hall

finish

Washington St

Devonshire St

Congress St

Stock Exchange Building

State St

Board of Trade Building

Custom House

India St

Central St

Broad St

Milk St

Hawes St

Water St

Liberty Square

Water St

Crab Alley

Kilby St

Water St

Milk St

Pearl St

Batterymarch St

Oliver St

Arch St

Devonshire St

Federal St

Congress St

Milk St

Post Office Square

Franklin St

Pearl St

Franklin St

Verizon Building

0   100   200   300 yards
0   100   200   300 meters

4 FINANCIAL DISTRICT: CRUISING THE CORRIDORS OF POWER

BOUNDARIES: **State St., Congress St., Franklin St., India St.**
DISTANCE: **Approx. 1 mile**
DIFFICULTY: **Easy**
PARKING: **Paid parking is available at 75 State St., Marketplace Center, and Post Office Square.**
PUBLIC TRANSIT: **State St. T Station on the Blue and Orange lines; busses 4, 92, and 93**

There was a time in the early and mid-19th century that Boston was the preeminent American city, and New York was playing catch-up. The remains of that financial powerhouse are located in the district of Boston just opposite the wharfs and south of Quincy Market. This walk ambles along avenues of skyscrapers, stops to enjoy a lovely midtown park oasis, and pokes into a few historic buildings before navigating some crooked back streets and hidden alleys to return to its starting place near the historic Old State House. Savor this walk in the spring, when the first warm days fill the park at Post Office Square and color bursts from the blooming tulips and daffodils.

● **Start at the State St. T Station. The large brick building with the gambrel roof and white steeple is the Old State House (established in 1713), which used to be the center of British rule in America and is now the oldest surviving public building in Boston. The first floor served as a merchant's hall and meeting place, while governmental meetings took place on the second floor.**

Stories about this place abound—from the fiery arguments of rebels to the Boston Massacre, which took place here on March 5, 1770. Look on the traffic island near Quaker Ln. for the plaque commemorating the five men who died in that riot. It all began when a British sentry had an altercation with a local youth. As it escalated, the commotion brought scores of sympathetic citizens to the boy's side and, eventually, eight more soldiers to back up the sentry. When the locals advanced on the Redcoats, shots were fired, and by the end of the night, five Boston civilians were dead.

Although the incident was minor and the mob may have been more to blame than the young soldiers, the altercation was quickly dubbed "the Bloody Massacre Perpetrated on King St." after Paul Revere distributed prints from an engraving he made showing his version the incident: well-formed lines of British infantry firing methodically into a loose cluster of civilians in broad daylight. Outraged revolutionaries used the event to whip the colonists into a fervor. It's little wonder, then, that the colonists used the Old State House for the first public reading of the Declaration of Independence. To find out more, consider taking one of the daily $5 tours offered by the Bostonian Society.

Before you get started, stop by the National Historical Park visitors center (look for the large banner), at 15 State St., which has bathrooms, some rudimentary exhibits, a gift shop, and plenty of helpful suggestions.

● Head east (toward the water) on State St. to the corner of State and Congress St.

● Turn right on Congress and follow it south to Franklin St. and Post Office Square. In the early 19th century, the building that was located at 12 Post Office Square (now merely a plaque) was the office of the *Liberator*, a newspaper founded in 1831 by abolitionist William Lloyd Garrison. The *Liberator* led the cry against slavery in antebellum New England. In the first edition, Garrison wrote, "I am in earnest. I will not equivocate. I will not excuse. I will not retreat a single inch—and I will be heard."

● At the corner of Franklin St. and Congress St., turn left to cross Congress and enter the Norman B. Leventhal Park at Post Office Square. This 1.7-acre green space—which features 125 different varieties of plants—is overshadowed on all sides by skyscrapers, but if you ignore the bustle of the Financial District, the park is a wonderful spot to take a break with a cappuccino or cup of tea at one of the tables around the pagoda. Wander north through the park along the birches, red oaks, and two giant arborvitaes on loan from the Arnold Arboretum. You'd never guess that under your feet are seven levels of parking that can hold 1,500 cars. Before the underground parking mecca (occasionally referred to as the "Garage Mahal") and the park were built, this was an ugly parking lot on street level. Now it's a privately owned but publicly accessible park. For a little bite or cappuccino for a break, head over to the Milk Street Cafe at the south end of the park—it's an outpost for the better known cafe around the corner on Milk St.

● From the southern edge of the park, cross over Franklin St. at the crosswalk and head for the Verizon Building at 185 Franklin. Built in 1947 as the New England Telephone Headquarters Building, this is one of the city's best remaining examples of late Art Deco architecture. Check out the small alcove off the lobby for its re-creation of Alexander Graham Bell's workshop, as well as a mural depicting the history of the telephone.

● Walk east on Franklin St. to 250 Franklin St. The Renaissance Revival-style Federal Reserve Building, is now the Langham Hotel. Walk into the lobby from the entrance facing Post Office Square to gawk at the high ceilings and polished marble, and then exit by the same door you came in, and continue on Franklin St.

● Turn left on Batterymarch St. and follow it to Liberty Square, where colonists pro-tested the 1765 Stamp Act (remember "no taxation without representation," from U.S. history class?). The square now boasts the striking Gyuri Hollosy statue com-memorating the student-led 1956 Hungarian Revolution, when thousands died and hundreds of thousands fled the country. Also check out the Neoclassical Appleton Building, at 10 Liberty Square. It boasts a variety of architectural styles, from the Italianate window on the first floor to the Ruskinian arch over the doors, and the Romanesque window on the top three floors.

● Retrace your steps to the eastern side of the square, between Water and Milk streets, and look for the small corridor called Crab Alley (reputed to get its name from a place where they sold, you guessed it, crabs)—one of the narrowest alleyways in all of Boston. Turn left on it to walk east to Broad St.

● Turn right on Broad and go one block.

● Turn left on Milk St. and follow it to India St.

● Turn left on India and walk to State St. On the corner of India and State streets is the Custom House, a Greek Revival-style building with simple lines and granite construction. Completed in 1849, this building helped solidify Boston's place as the cultural and commercial capital of New England. The 495-foot tower was added to the federal building in 1915, skirting local height restrictions and making it the tallest building in Boston for more than 30 years, until the John Hancock building was erected in Back Bay. The building is now owned by Marriott, which renovated it with high-end timeshare units.

● Turn left on State St. to return to the State St. T Station.

POINTS OF INTEREST

Old State House 206 Washington St., Boston, MA 02109, 617-720-1713

National Historical Park visitors center 15 State St., Boston, MA 02109, 617-242-5642

Milk Street Cafe Post Office Square at the intersection of Franklin and Congress streets, Boston, MA 02109, 617-542-3663

Langham Hotel 250 Franklin St., Boston, MA 02109, 617-451-1900

route summary

1. Start at the State St. T Station and head east on State.
2. Turn right on Congress St.
3. At the corner of Congress and Franklin streets, cross Congress to enter the park at Post Office Square and walk to the south end of the park.
4. Venture north through the park and then return south to cross Franklin St. and walk east on Franklin.

5.   Turn left on Batterymarch St. and continue northwest through Liberty Square.

6.   Retrace your steps to Crab Alley, and turn left.

7.   Turn right on Broad St.

8.   Turn left on Milk St.

9.   Turn left on India St.

10.   Turn left on State St. to return to the State St. T Station.

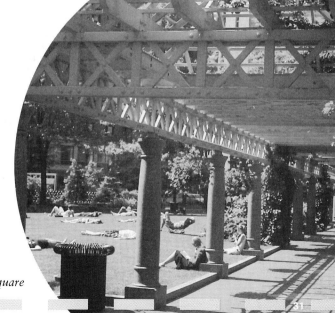

Post Office Square

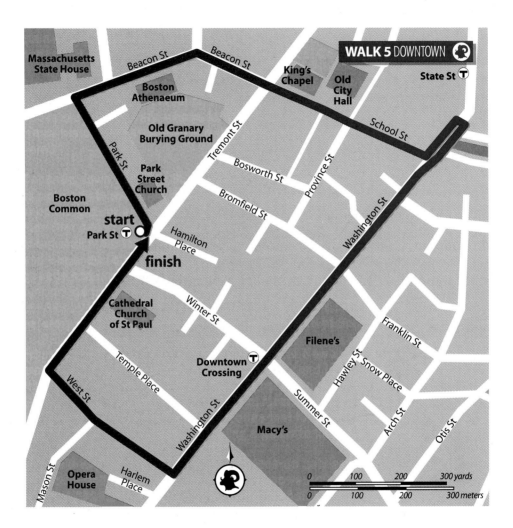

Massachusetts
State House

Beacon St

Beacon St

King's
Chapel

Old
City
Hall

State St Ⓣ

Boston
Athenaeum

School St

Old Granary
Burying Ground

Tremont St

Park St

Bosworth St

Province St

Park
Street
Church

Bromfield St

Washington St

Boston
Common

start
Park St Ⓣ ○

Hamilton
Place

finish

Cathedral
Church
of St Paul

Winter St

Franklin St

Filene's

Temple Place

Downtown
Crossing Ⓣ

Hawley St

Snow Place

West St

Washington St

Summer St

Arch St

Otis St

Mason St

Opera
House

Harlem
Place

Macy's

0   100   200   300 yards

0   100   200   300 meters

5 DOWNTOWN: CULTURE AND THE PARKER HOUSE ROLL

BOUNDARIES: **Tremont St., Beacon St., Washington St., and West St.**
DISTANCE: **Approx. 1¼ miles**
DIFFICULTY: **Easy**
PARKING: **Paid parking is available on Boylston St., at Boston Common Parking Garage, and on Washington St.**
PUBLIC TRANSIT: **Park St. T Station on the Green and Red lines; Downtown Crossing T Station; busses 42, 55, 92, and 93**

In the early 19th century, Boston was the undisputed cultural capital of the United States. Publishing houses, bookstores, and meeting spaces brimmed with revolutionary philosophy and radical literature. This walk mixes that wonderful historical pedigree with the vibrancy and energy that makes Boston such an interesting city today. And to fuel all the thinking this route stimulates, the trip ends at one of the nicest places in town for dinner.

You can save this walk for a late fall day when the blustery weather will make ducking into any of the charming stops along this tour all the more enticing.

● Start at the Park St. T Station. On September 1, 1898, at 6 AM, this station was crowded with more than 100 people who wanted to catch the first train of the morning, which also happened to be the first train of the subway's existence—and the first subway train ride in the history of the United States. It went from Park St. Station to what is now Government Center and helped relieve street-level congestion caused by the recent influx of cars.

Take a moment to look around the Park Street Church (1 Park St.), the site of abolitionist William Lloyd Garrison's first major antislavery speech in 1829. The church was also known as "Brimstone Corner" for the passionate preaching of its ministers (or perhaps because one of its ministers would sprinkle sulfur on the sidewalks to attract passersby). Today, it still functions as a church, and its distinctive white spire set atop the brick church is one of Boston's most recognizable landmarks, topping out at 217 feet.

- Walk north on Park to Beacon St., and cross Beacon (carefully, as this street is crammed with tour busses) to stand in front of the Massachusetts State House. Finished in 1798, the gold-domed edifice was designed by renowned Boston architect Charles Bulfinch. In a moment of irony, local wit Oliver Wendell Holmes declared the Massachusetts State House to be "the hub of the solar system," an epithet that quickly became a badge of pride for all of Boston. Today, "the Hub" is a favorite city nickname. You can catch a free tour of the inside. Be sure to look for the Sacred Cod, a 5-foot-long wooden fish that has hung in the Hall of Representatives for more than 200 years. Just don't try to leave the State House by the front door. That privilege is reserved for outgoing presidents and Massachusetts governors.

- Face the State House and turn right on Beacon St., following it east to 10½ Beacon. Built in 1849, the Boston Athenaeum is one of Boston's best places to read and research. Although it is a private library that requires a paid membership, guests are more than welcome to visit a few of the rooms or take an architectural tour on a Tuesday or Thursday. Just be careful of disturbing the ghosts. The writer Nathaniel Hawthorne ran into one while reading in the Athenaeum, and, out of respect for library decorum, Hawthorne did not make a sound. The ghost, meanwhile, could not address Hawthorne until spoken to (apparently, this is a rule governing ghostly conduct). According to Hawthorne, the two just waited silently for the other to speak until the ghost got frustrated and wandered off to find someone else to haunt.

- At the corner of Tremont St., continue southeast, where Beacon becomes School St., and duck into the famous Omni Parker House Hotel, at 60 School, for a snack. Established in 1855 and opened as the Parker House Hotel the very next year, this is one of the oldest and most prestigious addresses in town. The hotel has served as home to Charles Dickens and employed men like Ho Chi Minh and Malcolm X as busboys and waiters. Among the hotel's famous culinary creations are the Parker House roll, a fluffy dinner roll that was a household name toward the end of the 19th century, and the Boston cream pie, which has been fattening people for years. You can bite into these pieces of history in Parker's Restaurant or tip one back at The Last Hurrah Bar, where a young John F. Kennedy announced his run for U.S.

Congress in 1946. During the mid-19th century, the hotel hosted the Saturday Club, a monthly group of diners who came together to gab; the group included Ralph Waldo Emerson, Oliver Wendell Holmes, Nathaniel Hawthorne, and other major figures in American culture. The Grand Ballroom on the top floor affords wonderful views of Boston, from the Common to Government Center.

The King's Chapel and Old City Hall are opposite the hotel. Built in 1686, the grey stone King's Chapel was the first Anglican church in New England, and the Old City Hall served as the seat of Boston's government for more than a hundred years, until it was replaced by the modernistic City Hall in Government Center Plaza. This one, with its impressive columns and archways, is much more interesting to look at and offers tours.

Continue a few more steps on School St. to the former site of the Boston Latin School. Opened in 1635, Boston Latin was the first public school in the colonies. Although the school has long since moved to a location near the Museum of Fine Arts, you can find the shiny mosaic dedicated to the school embedded in the sidewalk near the statue of Benjamin Franklin, who was just one of its many famous students.

Continue along School to Washington St. The charming little two-story building on the north corner at 3 School St. was once the epicenter of American culture—it is the former home of Ticknor and Fields publishing company, and the Old Corner Bookstore. Ticknor and Fields published the works of important 19th-century American writers like Ralph Waldo Emerson, Henry David Thoreau, Nathaniel Hawthorne, and Henry Wadsworth Longfellow. When

Boston Athenaeum

in town, these literary icons would gather at the Old Corner Bookstore (Hawthorne even had a favorite chair in the corner) to discuss new developments in American letters. Although threatened by destruction, the building was saved in 1960 by the Historic Boston group. The building is now occupied by a jewelry store, but there is an interesting display about the building's history on the second floor.

If the Old Corner Bookstore represents the past, then the glass façade of the Borders bookstore across the street may represent the future, or at least the present. Its two stories of books, magazines, DVDs, and music provide enough material for endless browsing. There is also a bathroom on the second floor. Just in front of Borders is the *Irish Famine Memorial*, installed to commemorate the 150th anniversary of the Irish Famine. The bronze sculptures depict an Irish family, on their knees suffering in Ireland and striding forward in Boston toward a more hopeful future.

● From the corner of School and Washington streets, turn left to head northwest up Washington Street to 244 Washington. In 1872, the *Boston Globe* set up its headquarters

Back Story: Old Corner Bookstore

In the mid-19th century, every literary figure of record went to the Old Corner Bookstore. Nathaniel Hawthorne had his favorite secluded nook, where he could observe from the shadows, and Oliver Wendell Holmes was said to visit the bookstore at least once a day. Ticknor and Fields, which ran both the bookstore and a publishing house, was based out of the building as well. James Fields was noted for publishing such literary greats as Ralph Waldo Emerson, Nathaniel Hawthorne, and Oliver Wendell Holmes. He did, however, make one small mistake; he told Louisa May Alcott that she had no talent for writing and should stick to teaching.

here and was joined by five other newspapers, thus creating what was known as "Newspaper Row." In the glory days of the late 19th/early 20th centuries, each paper would write the day's headlines on large blackboards for people to read even before the papers went to press. After the *Globe* moved to Dorchester in 1958, the building was torn down and is now occupied by a parking lot. The peculiarly named Pi Alley refers to the Pi newsprint that was often discarded in the alley.

● Retrace your steps on Washington St. to the Old South Meeting House at 310 Washington—yet another historical hotspot. Imagine this early 18th-century brick building crammed with 7,000 people up in arms about a tax on tea, with everybody shouting and demanding that the tea on the ships in the harbor should not be unloaded. It's not surprising that later that night—on December 16, 1773—some 46 tons of tea leaves (or enough to brew 18,523,000 cups of tea) ended up in the water. The building's other claims to fame include being the site of Benjamin Franklin's baptism and the church of African-American poet Phyllis Wheatley. The building faced destruction in 1876, but Bostonians rallied to save Old South, and it is now a public museum as well as a civic space for lectures, meetings, concerts, and even weddings.

● Continue on Washington St. to a de facto pedestrian zone between Bromfield and West streets, where car traffic is severely limited and most everybody walks in the streets. This area has seen tremendous changes over the recent decades as retail giants like Filene's Basement and Macy's moved in and then, in some cases, moved back out. Local chain Filene's was a fixture on Washington St. for nearly a century (even the mayor of Boston shopped there). William Filene started a small shop in Salem in 1852 and had this Beaux Arts flagship store, designed by Daniel Burnham, built in 1912.

● Turn right on West St. At 15 West is the West Street Grille, the former home of Elizabeth Peabody's Bookshop, which served as a cultural center during the 1840s. Not only did writers and thinkers like Margaret Fuller, Nathaniel Hawthorne, and Ralph Waldo Emerson gather to talk, but Charles Ripley drew up his plans for the utopian society Brook Farm here. In 1842, Elizabeth Peabody became the country's first woman publisher when she published the transcendentalist journal *The Dial* from the bookshop.

Before you go in, take a moment to browse the shelves of the Brattle Bookshop, next door, at 9 West St. Brattle Books has been in operation (although not on West St. the whole time) since 1825. It has a dizzying array of used and antiquarian books, and the proprietors, Ken Gloss and Joyce Kosofsky, are nationally recognized experts on antiquarian books. It is worth a few moments perusing the overloaded shelves inside or the rolling bins of books that fill the adjacent alley. The selection of books on New England is particularly enticing.

Once your hunger becomes unbearable, go into the West Street Grille for lunch or dinner. The charm of the old building is a delightful complement to the white starched table linen and dishes like the chicken salad club "West Street style." While it is possible to just drop by for a meal, reservations are a good idea, particularly on busy Friday or Saturday nights. Be sure to note the green plaque to the left of the door. It tells the story of Elizabeth Peabody's bookstore and its role in shaping 19th-century American culture.

● Continue on West to Tremont St., which borders the Boston Common.

● Cross Tremont to the visitors center, and then turn right to follow Tremont to your starting point at the Park St. T Station.

POINTS OF INTEREST

Park Street Church 1 Park St., Boston, MA 02108, 617-523-3383

Massachusetts State House 1 Beacon St., Boston, MA 02133, 617-727-3676

Boston Athenaeum 10½ Beacon St., Boston, MA 02108, 617-227-0270

Omni Parker House Hotel 60 School St., Boston, MA 02108, 617-227-8600

King's Chapel 58 Tremont St., Boston, MA 02108, 617-523-1749

Old Corner Bookstore Building 3 School St., Boston, MA 02108

Old South Meeting House 310 Washington St., Boston, MA 02108, 617-482-6439

West Street Grille 15 West St., Boston, MA 02110, 617-423-0300

Brattle Books 9 West St., Boston, MA 02110, 617-542-0210

route summary

1. From the Park St. T Station, head north on Park.
2. Turn right on **Beacon St.** and follow it until it becomes School St. at intersection of Tremont St.
3. Continue southeast on School St.
4. Turn left on Washington St. and follow it to 244 Washington St.
5. Retrace your steps on **Washington St.** and walk south to West St.
6. Turn right on West St.
7. Turn right on Tremont St. to return to the Park St. T Station.

Irish Famine Memorial

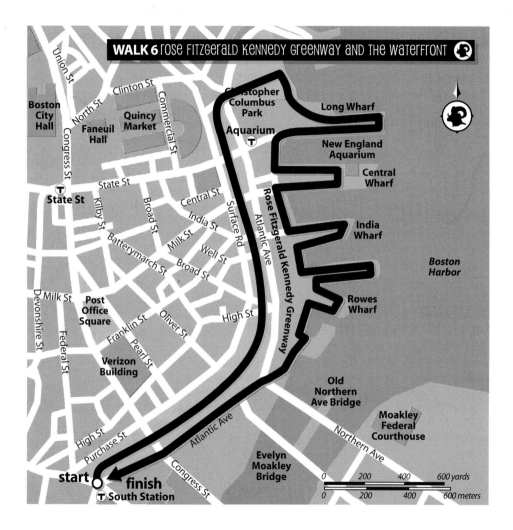

Union St

Clinton St

North St

Commercial St

Boston City Hall

Congress St

Faneuil Hall

Quincy Market

Christopher Columbus Park

Long Wharf

Aquarium

New England Aquarium

State St

State St

Kilby St

Central St

Broad St

India St

Surface Rd

Atlantic Ave

Rose Fitzgerald Kennedy Greenway

Central Wharf

India Wharf

Batterymarch St

Milk St

Well St

Broad St

Boston Harbor

Devonshire St

Milk St

Post Office Square

High St

Rowes Wharf

Federal St

Franklin St

Oliver St

Pearl St

Verizon Building

Old Northern Ave Bridge

Moakley Federal Courthouse

High St

Purchase St

Atlantic Ave

Northern Ave

start

Congress St

finish

Evelyn Moakley Bridge

South Station

0	200	400	600 yards
0	200	400	600 meters

6 rose FITZGeralD KenneDy Greenway anD THe waTerFronT: DIGGING THe BIG DIG anD walking THe waTerFronT

BOUNDARIES: Summer St., Surface Rd., Atlantic Ave., Boston Harbor
DISTANCE: Approx. 2½ miles
DIFFICULTY: Easy
PARKING: Paid parking is available on Summer St., at the Rowes Wharf Garage, at the Sargent's Wharf Garage, at the aquarium's Harbor Garage, and at Lewis Wharf Parking.
PUBLIC TRANSIT: South Station T Station on the Red Line; busses 6, 7, 448, 449, and 459

This may be the most exciting walk in Boston. For decades, this area was the dirty underbelly of a highway. Then for many years, it was merely another construction site in a city besieged by bulldozers. Now, this parkway, bordered by Atlantic Ave. on the east and the unimaginatively named Surface Rd. on the west, is a 5-acre greenway reuniting Boston with its long estranged waterfront. Boasting everything from interactive water fountains to open green spaces, the Rose Fitzgerald Kennedy Greenway is a major draw for this part of the city. This tour goes out along the greenway and returns along the Harborwalk, a series of connected paths that lines most of Boston's waterfront, from Dorchester to East Boston.

This is a great walk for a summer afternoon, when the greenway buzzes people and the harbor rings with the sounds of boats and summer concerts.

● **Start inside the South Station T Station. Built in 1898 to be the largest train station in the world, South Station is Boston's main terminal for trains heading to New York City, Washington, D.C., and beyond. Scheduled for demolition in 1970 (they had even begun dismantling the once grand structure), South Station was rescued by a local group that managed to get it listed on the National Register of Historic Places. In 1984, the Massachusetts Bay Transportation Authority dumped nearly $200 million into renovation and restored the station to its former glory. Today, it has the wonderful feel of a train station, with a wide-open foyer and an enormous clacking sign proclaiming train arrivals and departures. South Station also has the train station** standards—newsstands, cafes, and ice-cream shops, and there are bathrooms along the north wall of the terminal.

● Exit the train station through the main doors to the corner of Atlantic Ave. and Summer St. Cross to the north side of the intersection and begin walking northeast through the Rose Fitzgerald Kennedy Greenway, whose Boston native namesake was the matriarch of the Kennedy clan and mother of John, Robert, and Edward.

From South Station, the first plazas you enter are the Dewey Square Parks. These open, landscaped sections with meandering footpaths offer a lovely stroll as you work your way northeast across Congress St. and past Seaport Blvd. and Northern Ave. until you arrive at the plaza between Oliver and High streets. Although this section is currently an open green space, work will begin in 2012 for the new Center for Arts and Culture, a performance and gallery space.

● Just past this parcel is the entrance to the Wharf District Parks, which begin at High Street (just opposite Rowes Wharf). The plaza offers a peek into Boston's maritime heritage, with granite seawall stones from nearby Rumney Marsh, nautical sculptures, and machine that creates a "harbor fog" mist that is illuminated at night.

● Continue north to the next plaza, between India and Milk streets. Built on a "great room" model, this section's open green spaces and seating are designed for festivals, fairs, concerts, and performances.

● The next plaza, between State and Milk streets, features the Landmark Rings Fountain, which shoots choreographed spouts of water more than 30 feet into the air. After looking up, look down, where, beginning in 2008, workers will install engraved pavers into a section called the "Mother's Walk."

● Continue north to the Walk to the Sea, a plaza bisecting the greenway connecting Faneuil Hall with Long Wharf. At the center of this park is the Harbor Park Pavilion, Boston's gateway to the 34 harbor islands in the Boston Bay that were designated as a national park in 1996. This also marks the northern edge of the Wharf District Parks.

- Where Atlantic Ave. comes in from the North End and crosses into the park, turn right to enter Christopher Columbus Park. This park was slated for a large parking garage in the 1960s but plans were discarded after an intense local outcry against the garage. Expanded and renovated as part of the Big Dig, it is particularly impressive in the spring, when the tulips near the playground are in full bloom. Flower lovers should also make sure to stroll by the Rose Kennedy Rose Garden.

- Exit the park on the southern edge (toward the Marriott Hotel, which has bathrooms and large maritime paintings on the second floor) to access the Harborwalk and the Marriott Hotel. The Harborwalk's namesake is a nonprofit group that has been working to create walking paths along the waterfront from Dorchester through East Boston.

- From the hotel, follow the wooden pathway along the northern edge of Long Wharf to the wharf's end, where you can look through the telescopes at the inner harbor. If you need a little directional help, try finding the compass rose made from pink stone set in the ground. At one time, up to 50 large shipping vessels would dock at the wharf, and the wharf itself would be packed high with cargo.

- From the end of Long Wharf, continue following the Harborwalk (look for the blue signs with a white sailboat) south as it meanders along the shoreline. The next wharf you come to is Central Wharf, home to the New England Aquarium. The aquarium specializes in harbor seals, penguins, barracuda, giant sea turtles, and has what was for a while the largest indoor shark tank. It's worth an afternoon stop if you have kids.

Long Wharf

If you don't want to invest in the full experience, stop at the seal tank to watch the animals frolic; it's free and entertaining.

- From the aquarium, continue south on the Harborwalk to India Wharf. Here you'll find a set of four sculptures designed by David von Schlegell. Stand in the middle of them and try to make out whether the forms are from land or sea. If floating sculptures are more to your taste, turn around and look over the harbor, especially to your right. During the summer months, these berths are usually taken by some pretty fancy yachts.

- Continue down Harborwalk to Rowes Wharf. The stone archway of the Boston Harbor Hotel is worth stopping for, as is the lobby, which holds a collection of more than 90 antique maps of Boston and New England. For a view of the harbor, head up to the ninth-floor observatory, Foster's Rotunda. In the summer, the patios outside the hotel are rocking with a floating dock brought in for free concerts and movies.

- Continue along the Harborwalk toward the Old Northern Ave. Bridge, and go up the stairs to return to street level. At the corner of the bridge and Atlantic Ave. is James Hook and Company, a family-run fish store that's been on the waterfront since 1925. Sidle up to the large front window for a good look at their "lobbies" and other denizens of the deep.

- With James Hook behind you, face north and turn left on Atlantic to return to the South Station T Station.

POINTS OF INTEREST

South Station T Station 245 Summer St., Boston, MA 02110, 617-222-5215

Rose Fitzgerald Kennedy Greenway Along Atlantic Ave. between Summer and State streets, Boston, MA 02109, 617-292-0020

Christopher Columbus Park Corner of Cross St. and Atlantic Ave., Boston, MA 02109, 617-635-4505

Boston Marriott Hotel 296 State St., Boston, MA 02109, 617-227-0800

New England Aquarium Central Wharf, Boston, MA 02110, 617-973-5200

Boston Harbor Hotel 70 Rowes Wharf, Boston, MA 02110, 617-439-7000

James Hook and Company 15–17 Northern Ave., Boston, MA 02210, 617-423-5500

ROUTE SUMMARY

1. Begin at the South Station T Station.
2. Walk northeast on the Rose Fitzgerald Kennedy Greenway toward Christopher Columbus Park.
3. Turn right to walk through Columbus Park, to its southern edge.
4. From Columbus Park, join the Harborwalk behind the Marriott Hotel on Long Wharf.
5. Follow the Harborwalk south along the waterfront to the Old Northern Ave. Bridge.
6. Climb the stairs to reach street level and turn left on Atlantic Ave. to return to the South Station T Station.

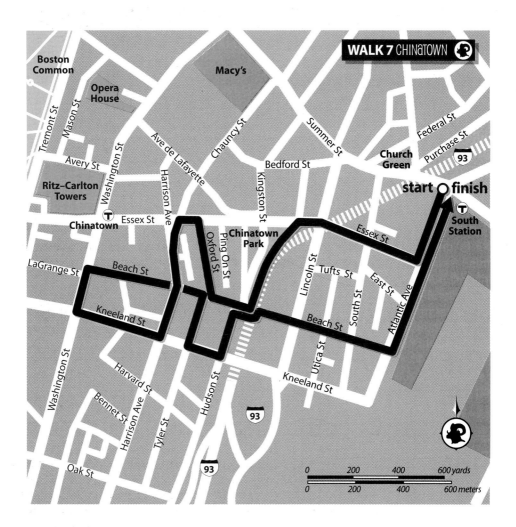

7 CHINATOWN: NOODLES AND MOON CAKE WALK

BOUNDARIES: Atlantic Ave., Kneeland St., Washington St., Essex St.

DISTANCE: Approx. 1¼ miles

DIFFICULTY: Easy

PARKING: There are parking lots at South Station T Station and on Essex St.

PUBLIC TRANSIT: South Station T Station on the Orange Line; busses 3, 6, 7, 11, 500, 501, 504, 505, 553, 554, 556, and 558

Looks can be deceiving. Boston's Chinatown may look small, but it is the third largest Chinatown in the country (behind only San Francisco and New York City). While perhaps overshadowed by the city's better known Italian North End or the Irish neighborhoods south of Boston, this little gem offers great tightly packed streets, colorful architecture, and an intriguing history going back hundreds of years. The short distances of this walk allow plenty of time for window-shopping and sampling from any of the Cambodian, Vietnamese, and Cantonese restaurants crammed along the streets.

Like the tour of the North End, this is a great one for the winter, when steaming bowls of soup from Pho Pasteur or a warm cake from the Hin Shing Bakery will make the contrast with the chilly weather even more delicious.

- Begin at the South Station T Station. From the main doors at the corner of Atlantic Ave. and Summer St., turn left to head south on Atlantic one short block to Essex St. (you can also access Essex from the side entrance of South Station).

- Turn right on Essex and follow it two blocks to the start of Chinatown Park.

- Carefully cross Surface Rd. at the crosswalk and turn left to walk southwest through Chinatown Park, a nearly acre-size expanse that hosts celebrations and activities like the Chinese New Year, lantern festivals, and outdoor markets with cafe dining and puppet theaters. It is also the first section of the Rose Fitzgerald Kennedy Greenway. Created with significant input from local residents and experts in Asian landscape design, the park follows feng shui ideals of balance and harmony and makes use of traditional Chinese design elements such as bamboo, water, stone, and gates.

At the northern end is one of the biggest draws, a large sail sculpture that is illuminated with red at night. Just beyond, on the right, is a waterfall with a large bamboo screen. Both sides of the winding path are lined with bamboo, willow, Chinese cherry trees, azaleas, gingko, and peonies. All of these were chosen because of their beauty and cultural significance.

The path widens near the Chinatown gates, in front of which is a tile pattern in the ground reminiscent of a Chinese checkerboard. The design was created by California artist May Sun and, if you look closely, you can see a map of Boston centered on the area near Chinatown.

Turn and look up at the Chinatown gates. A gift from the Taiwanese government in 1982, these gates are inscribed with the message, "Everything under the sky is for the people."

● Facing the Chinatown gates at the corner of Beach and Hudson streets, proceed ahead (west) on Beach. You are now entering Chinatown proper. Originally known as South Cove (like so many places in Boston, this was shoreline before it was filled in), this area first attracted Chinese immigrants in the late 19th century, as they came to work in the nearby garment district.

The first tiny alleyway on the right leads to Ping On St. In the late 19th century, Chinese workers were brought to Boston to work in the textile industries, and they first lived in a collection of tents along what is now known as Ping On St. Later, as their numbers grew, the immigrants built permanent houses throughout the neighborhood and farther down into South Boston. However, the construction of the interstate, coupled with economic development, condensed Chinatown into the compact neighborhood it is today.

● Turn right on Oxford St. In 1761, the intersection of Oxford St. and Beach St.—at the time a wharf—was the site where a young girl kidnapped from Africa's west coast was purchased by Susanna Wheatley, wife of a prosperous Boston merchant John

Wheatley. The young girl was given the name of the ship that brought her to America and the name of the family that bought her, making her name Phillis Wheatley. Later in her life, Wheatley became America's first published African-American poet, and her life and work is celebrated in a monument on Commonwealth Ave.

- Bear left at the first cluster of trees to duck down the tiny alleyway of Oxford Pl., where you can view the Chinatown heritage mural. Titled *Travelers in an Autumn Landscape*, the mural, done in 1980 by Wenli Zen and Zuio Yuan, is a copy of a Qing Dynasty painting by Yun Wang that formerly hung in the Museum of Fine Arts in the Back Bay Fens.

- Retrace your steps to Oxford St., and turn left to continue to Essex St.

- Turn left on Essex and continue to Harrison Ave.

- Turn left on Harrison Ave. As you journey down Harrison, you can stop by the Eldo Cake House Bakery, at 36 Harrison, if you are in the mood for a little snack. If you are big on hunger and short on cash, try the Hong Kong Eatery at 79 Harrison Ave. for pork and rice.

- Turn right on Kneeland St. and continue to Washington St.

- Turn right on Washington and stop at Pho Pasteur, at the corner of Washington and Beach streets, for what many say is the best place in Boston for Vietnamese noodles. At $5 to $8 per bowl, it's also an affordable meal.

A street vendor in Chinatown

- Turn right on Beach St., Chinatown's main thoroughfare and a street so wide it feels much like a town square.

- Turn right on Tyler St., whose brightly colored storefronts advertise everything from electronics to freshly skinned chickens. At the corner of Beach St. and Tyler St. is the Peach Farm restaurant, another great place to ignore the English menu and order what you see others having.

  Also check out the intricate balconies, reminiscent of Chinese tea balconies, above the Lucky House Seafood Restaurant, at 10 Tyler St.

- Turn left on Kneeland St. and continue to Hudson St.

- Turn left on Hudson and just before the Chinatown gates, stop in for a pastry at Hin Shing Bakery, on the corner of Hudson and Beach streets. The mixed nut moon cake is divine, especially if it's still hot. Get your pastry to go and bring it across Hudson to eat in Chinatown Park.

- After your snack, go to the intersection of Hudson and Beach St. and walk east on Beach, crossing Surface Rd. Although it may not look like it today, this section is called the Leather District, for clothing warehouses and manufacturers that once lined the streets here. Today many of those warehouses have been converted into condos and office buildings.

- Turn left on Atlantic Ave. to return to the South Station T Station.

POINTS OF INTEREST

Chinatown Park Corner of Essex St. and Surface Rd., Boston, MA 02111
Eldo Cake House Bakery 36 Harrison Ave., Boston, MA 02111, 617-350-7977
Hong Kong Eatery 79 Harrison Ave., Boston, MA 02111, 617-423-0838
Pho Pasteur 682 Washington St., Boston, MA 02111, 617-482-7467
Peach Farm 4 Tyler St., Boston, MA 02111, 617-482-3332
Lucky House Seafood Restaurant 10 Tyler St., Boston, MA 02111, 617-338-9038
Hin Shing Bakery 67 Beach St., Boston, MA 02111, 617-451-1162

route summary

1. Start at South Station T Station and walk south on Atlantic Ave.
2. Turn right on Essex St.
3. Cross Surface Rd. and turn left to walk southwest through Chinatown Park to the Chinatown gates at corner of Beach and Hudson streets.
4. Turn right on Beach St.
5. Turn right on Oxford St.
6. Bear left on Oxford Pl.
7. Return to Oxford St. and turn left.
8. Turn left on Essex St.
9. Turn left on Harrison Ave.
10. Turn right on Kneeland St.
11. Turn right on Washington St.
12. Turn right on Beach St.
13. Turn right on Tyler St.
14. Turn left on Kneeland St.
15. Turn left on Hudson St.
16. Turn right on Beach St.
17. Turn left on Atlantic Ave. to return to South Station T Station.

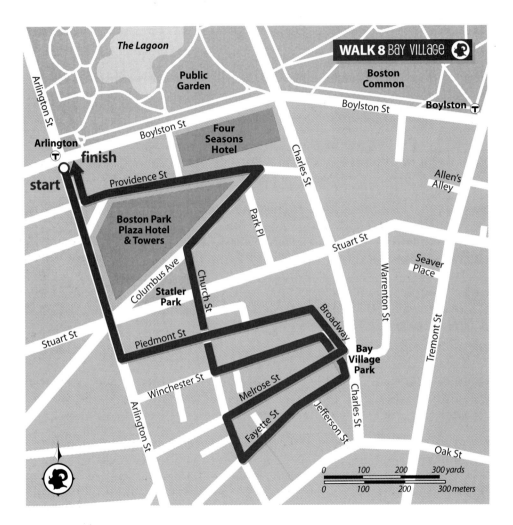

The Lagoon

Public Garden

Boston Common

Boylston St

Boylston

Arlington St

Boylston St

Four Seasons Hotel

Allen's Alley

Arlington

finish

start

Providence St

Park Pl

Charles St

Boston Park Plaza Hotel & Towers

Stuart St

Columbus Ave

Seaver Place

Statler Park

Church St

Warrenton St

Tremont St

Stuart St

Piedmont St

Broadway

Bay Village Park

Winchester St

Melrose St

Charles St

Arlington St

Fayette St

Jefferson St

Oak St

| 0 | 100 | 200 | 300 yards |
| 0 | 100 | 200 | 300 meters |

8 Bay Village: Quiet Cobblestones and a Fiery Tragedy

BOUNDARIES: **Boylston St., Arlington St., Fayette St., Charles St.**
DISTANCE: **Approx. 1 mile**
DIFFICULTY: **Easy**
PARKING: **Although there is very little on-street parking, a parking garage is available at the corner of Columbus Ave. and Providence St. (across the street from Finale).**
PUBLIC TRANSPORTATION: **Arlington T Station on the Green Line; busses 9, 39, and 55**

It has been known by many names—the Church Street District, South Cove, and Kerry Village—but Bay Village is the name that endured. By whatever name, this six-block neighborhood is one of Boston's best-kept secrets. Stumbling into Bay Village can feel a bit like wandering onto a 1930s movie set. The well-kept brownstones and cobblestone streets make the neighborhood seem like a smaller, less-ornate version of Beacon Hill, which in fact it is. Wandering among the quiet, tree-lined avenues, you may have a hard time believing you are still in the heart of Boston, just steps away from the Boston Common.

With its lovely houses and postage-stamp parks, this quiet neighborhood is perfectly suited for a summer evening's stroll.

● **Begin at the Arlington T Station and proceed south (away from the Boston Common) on Arlington St. As is the case in many places throughout Boston, Arlington St. was once waterfront before Back Bay was filled in.**

After two blocks, stop at the intersection of Columbus Ave. and Arlington St. to see the "Castle" (101 Arlington St.), the former armory and headquarters for the First Corps of Cadets. The First Corps was a late 19th-century civilian military group that rose in response to the riots following the depression in the 1870s. Today, the upscale steak restaurant Smith & Wollensky has renovated the gun room and others into fine dining rooms. The medieval castle is listed on the National Register of Historic Places.

Back Story: Coconut Grove Fire

In 1942, Boston was brimming with soldiers on leave, hardworking immigrants, and movie stars. The Coconut Grove nightclub was one place they all went. Built as a tropical paradise, this huge club featured palm trees and a roof that could be rolled back for a magical night dancing under the stars. It could host nearly a thousand people.

When a young couple unscrewed a light bulb for a bit of privacy on the cold evening of November 28, 1942, a busboy was told to screw it back in. Unable to find the socket in the dim light, the busboy lit a match and inadvertently sparked one of the artificial palm fronds in the overhead canopy. At first, there was laughter, as waiters tried to douse the flames with seltzer water while the piano player played "Bell Bottom Trousers." But then the flames reached a stairwell and shot up to the main floor where Mickey Alpert's band was about to begin its second set. The fire spread quickly and people rushed for the exits, but, unfortunately, many of the doors were locked and the revolving doors were jammed with the crush of people.

The fire eventually killed 492 people and required 187 firefighters, 26 engine companies, and an entire water tower to put it out. It was the city's deadliest event at the time. However, as a result of the tragedy, techniques for treating burn victims were developed, and cities across the country tightened building codes to require lighted exit signs, doors that open outward, and revolving doors flanked by conventional doors.

● Proceed another block down Arlington, turn left on Piedmont St. to head east toward Broadway, and stop at 17 Piedmont to read the plaque set into the brick walkway on the north side of the road. It commemorates the 1942 Coconut Grove nightclub fire, which killed 492 people in less than 15 minutes. The emergency doors were locked, trapping the people inside. The Bay Village Neighborhood Association placed the plaque here in 1992, on the 50th anniversary of the fire.

● Turn right on Broadway and continue two blocks to Melrose St.

● Turn right on Melrose and follow it to Church St. The architects and builders who did much of the work on Beacon Hill made their homes in Bay Village, so there are a lot of similarities between the homes on Beacon Hill and many of the Greek Revival townhouses along Melrose. Here, you will see the same bow fronts and bay windows, the same fanlights and gambrels over the doors, and some of the same ironwork and brick patterns—only smaller and more modest versions than the ones at their Beacon Hill cousins. One of the main builders was Ephraim Marsh, who constructed approximately 300 homes throughout the Boston area in the 1820s. He lived one block over, at 1 Fayette St., in a house that he built.

● Turn left on Church St. and go two blocks to the corner of Church and Fayette St., to a tiny sandwich shop at 12 Church. Rachel's Kitchen is a local favorite, and it's easy to see why: friendly service, fresh ingredients, and a sandwich called "I'll Have What He's Having" (other sandwiches include the "Big Bad Wolf" and "a.k.'s easy caprese"). You may have to fight for a place to eat it, though—there is limited counter space inside and only a couple of tables outside. If the weather is nice, grab your sandwich and head for the Bay Village Park at the corner of Fayette and Broadway.

● Turn left on Fayette St. to head east. Fayette was named for the Revolutionary War hero Marquis de Lafayette, a close friend and compatriot of George Washington. Lafayette received a hero's welcome in Boston in 1842, the year Fayette St. was laid out. The street boasts several lovely, Federal-style row houses based on the English Neoclassic design (look for American eagle motifs). Note the lower windows of the houses as well as the arches that lead to stables in the back on the right side. In the

Church Street

mid-19th century, when the city began filling in what is now Back Bay, the streets in Bay Village were raised by 12 to 18 feet, and now the windows are well below street level. House 30A is a good example of this.

- At the end of Fayette, turn left to enter the Bay Village Park, a small, quiet space with benches and plants maintained by the Bay Village Neighborhood Association and the Boston Parks and Recreation Department.

- Exit the park on the north side, at the corner of Broadway and Melrose St. and walk north on Broadway for one block.

- Turn left on Winchester St. Some of the buildings along this street were once warehouses for the major film companies that produced newsreels in Bay Village during the first half of the 20th century. These buildings were specially built to withstand the weight of thousands of newsreels and to withstand fire.

- Turn right on Church St. At the intersection of Church and Stuart streets, turn around and look back down Church to Bay Village; you can almost see the quiet street fading away as you enter busy downtown again. No matter, if you forge ahead, you will come to one of the best ideas in Boston: dessert as a meal.

- Continue on Church and cross Stuart at the crosswalk, passing by the park and continuing on to Columbus Ave.

- Turn right on Columbus Ave. and walk to the corner of Columbus and Park Plaza. On your right is a statue of Abraham Lincoln standing over a freed African-American man. The statue was given to the city in 1879 by Moses Kimball, a Boston businessman and associate of P.T. Barnum.

- To rest from your labors, turn around and cross Columbus Ave. to the triangular restaurant Finale, a high-end dessert spot (they do have a light dinner menu as well) that's an experience in itself. Just try a sip of the hot chocolate, and you'll have a tough time leaving. If that doesn't get you, the Molten Chocolate Cake will. Get a booth by one of the windows that wrap around this sweet spot, and you may be here all afternoon.

- Once you do leave, waddle around the corner to the left and head west on Providence St. The Four Seasons is on the right, and the Boston Park Plaza is on the left.

- Unless you've booked a room at either of those upscale crashing places, turn right on Arlington St. to return to the Arlington T Station and your own less expensive bed.

POINTS OF INTEREST

Smith & Wollensky 101 Arlington St., Boston, MA 02116, 617-423-1112

Rachel's Kitchen 12 Church St., Boston, MA 02116, 617-423-3447

Bay Village Park Corner of Fayette St. and Broadway, Boston, MA 02116

Finale 1 Columbus Ave., Boston, MA 02116, 617-423-3184

ROUTE SUMMARY

1. Begin at the Arlington T Station and head south on Arlington St.
2. Turn left on Piedmont St.
3. Turn right on Broadway.
4. Turn right on Melrose St.
5. Turn left on Church St.
6. Turn left on Fayette St.
7. Turn left to enter the Bay Village Park.
8. Exit the park on the north side and walk north on Broadway.
9. Turn left on Winchester St.
10. Turn right on Church St.
11. Turn right on Columbus Ave.
12. Take a sharp left on Providence St.
13. Turn right on Arlington St. to return to the Arlington T Station.

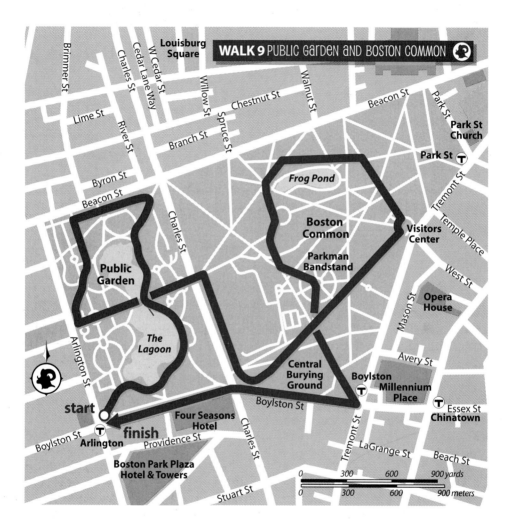

WALK 9 PUBLIC GARDEN AND BOSTON COMMON

Brimmer St

W Cedar St

Cedar Lane Way

Charles St

Louisburg Square

Willow St

Spruce St

Chestnut St

Walnut St

Beacon St

Park St

Park St Church

Park St (T)

Tremont St

Temple Place

Lime St

River St

Branch St

Byron St

Beacon St

Charles St

Frog Pond

Boston Common

Visitors Center

West St

Public Garden

Parkman Bandstand

Mason St

Opera House

The Lagoon

Arlington St

Central Burying Ground

Boylston (T)

Avery St

Millennium Place

Essex St (T) Chinatown

start

Boylston St

Boylston St

finish

Arlington (T)

Four Seasons Hotel

Providence St

Charles St

Boylston St

Tremont St

LaGrange St

Beach St

Boston Park Plaza Hotel & Towers

Stuart St

| 0 | 300 | 600 | 900 yards |
| 0 | 300 | 600 | 900 meters |

9 PUBLIC GARDEN AND BOSTON COMMON: AN UNCOMMON GARDEN

BOUNDARIES: Boylston St., Tremont St., Park St., Beacon St., Arlington St.
DISTANCE: Approx. 2 miles
DIFFICULTY: Easy
PARKING: Boston Common Parking Garage on Charles St.
PUBLIC TRANSPORTATION: Arlington T Station on the Green Line; busses 43 and 55

Although Boston Common and Public Garden were established 200 years apart (Boston Common in 1634 and the Public Garden in 1837), and they are separated by busy Charles St., these two public green spaces are linked in many people's minds. Combined, they form 75 acres of green fields, winding paths, waterways, and gardens, but they also offer two different experiences. The Public Garden is more formal, with Victorian garden designs featuring brass nametags on the trees, while the Common has more utilitarian offerings like bandstands, skating rinks, ball fields, and playgrounds.

This walk is perfect for late April and early May, before the hordes of summer tourists arrive, but right when the legions of silky tulips in every imaginable shade bloom along the paths. One note peculiar to this walk: Since the paths are not named, the directions provided here rely more on north, south, east, and west and navigation by sight. Not to worry, though, all the paths lead somewhere interesting, and people are more than happy to help with directions.

● **Start at the Arlington T Station and enter the Public Garden at the corner of Arlington and Boylston streets.**

● **Bear right around the lagoon to work your way toward the swan boats landing on the east side of the lagoon. These graceful, wooden, 30-foot pontoon boats have large, fiberglass swan figurines attached to the stern. Robert Paget, who designed the boats based on ones he had seen in a production of Richard Wagner's *Lohengrin*, floated the first boats in 1877. The business is still run by members of the Paget family. For less than $3, you can get a 15-minute, figure-eight ride around the**

3-acre lagoon, while the captain propels the boats from a bike seat attached to a paddle wheel.

● From the lagoon, meander along the paths toward the northeast corner of the Garden, at Charles and Beacon streets. Just before the busy intersection, you encounter a mother goose and her eight goslings, all in a row. Fans of Robert McCloskey's 1941 classic children's story, *Make Way for Ducklings*, will need no introduction to the brass figures of Mrs. Mallard and Jack, Kack, Lack, Mack, Nack, Ouack, Pack, and Quack. Nancy Schon's brass sculptures were introduced into the Public Garden in 1987 and have been polished to a bright sheen by countless hugs and kisses ever since.

● From the ducklings, head southwest along the north edge of the lagoon toward the entrance by Commonwealth Ave. Along the way, you pass a 40-foot granite and marble monument dedicated to the discovery of the anesthesia ether by Boston physicians. (As anybody who has ever had dental surgery can attest, this was a medical advance worthy of a monument.) Then wind over to the central gates of the Garden, at the intersection of Commonwealth Ave. and Arlington St.

Standing at the Arlington St. gates, you are face to face (well, sort of, he's kind of tall) with George Washington. The Thomas Ball sculpture of the first U.S. president riding his horse into battle was erected in the Public Garden in 1869. This area is one of the best spots in the Garden for a springtime photo of rows upon rows of tulips, with the Massachusetts Statehouse and downtown in the background.

● After this photo op, walk east and cross over the stone bridge by the swan boats and through the Garden to Charles St.

Standing on Charles St., between the Public Garden and Boston Common, you can note some of the differences between the two: The Garden has fences and gates; the Common does not. The Common is open and wide, while the Garden is more shaded and hidden. Both are usually full of activity and people, but the Common is less intimate: There are vendors hawking all sorts of goods; large-scale theatrical performances, concerts, and demonstrations; and children playing in playgrounds and teams playing baseball.

● Cross Charles St. and enter Boston Common. Turn right (south) and take the path that parallels Charles to edge of the park on Boylston St. In the corner of the Common, near the intersection of Boylston and Charles, is the Central Burying Ground, where soldiers from the Battle of Bunker Hill were laid to rest.

● From the burying ground, take the path leading northeast for a long, straight shot to the visitors center, at 147 Tremont. In addition to information about the Boston area, the center features bathrooms, T-shirt vendors, tour guides in 18th-century costumes, snacks, and often performers gathering a crowd in the wide plaza out front. If nobody is juggling bowling pins from a unicycle while holding a flaming torch in his mouth, there's still plenty to see here. One of the best times to be at the plaza is when there is enough quiet to study the sculptures *Learning*, *Industry*, and *Religion*, which adorn the plaza. To wit, the statue titled *Learning* features a young man astride a globe imprinted with mystical characters and reading a book.

● Walk to the back side of the visitors center and take the middle of the three paths that branch out toward the former site of the "Great Elm." The elm—which toppled in 1876 after it was damaged by a severe windstorm—served as the public gallows during the 17th century.

● For something a bit lighter, continue west along the same path to the Frog Pond, a water park in the summer and an ice-skating rink in the winter. The pond (no longer home to chirping amphibians) has long been a favorite among Bostonians. Nonetheless, the poet Edgar Allan Poe, who was born nearby in Bay Village, used the name to signify Boston's cultural insignificance, calling the city "Frogpondium." It's a slight Boston has yet to forgive.

Public Garden gates

BaCK STORY: WaLKING WITH WHITMaN

Boston Common has been the site of papal masses, rock concerts, baseball games, public hangings, Shakespeare plays, military training, cow grazing, pranks, shenanigans, and public spectacles aplenty.

However, my favorite story involves just two men walking the paths and talking. In February of 1867, Ralph Waldo Emerson and Walt Whitman ambled along the paths and talked about poetry. Well, Emerson talked, and Whitman had to listen. The topic of discussion was Whitman's poetry, which Emerson found a little racy. Under a barrage of logic and pleading, Whitman saw Emerson's point, but in the end he decided not to change a thing.

Here's how Whitman recounted the story:

During those two hours, he was the talker and I the listener. It was an argument-statement, reconnoitering, review, attack, and pressing home . . . of all that could be said against that part (and a main part) in the construction of one of my poems, "Children of Adam" . . . I could never hear the points better put—and then I felt down in my soul the clear and unmistakable conviction to disobey all and pursue my own way.

Although Emerson was unsuccessful in persuading Whitman to change his poetry, they went off and had a lovely dinner together, and Whitman went on to become one of the most important poets America has ever produced.

- From Frog Pond, turn left and head west down the path to the Soldiers and Sailors Monument atop Flagstaff Hill. The monument, a tribute to those who fought in the Civil War, affords wonderful views of the city and is a starting place for wintertime sledding. It was created in 1877 by the Irish brothers Martin, Joseph, and James Milmore. See if you can identify the historical figures in the bronze reliefs.

- From Flagstaff Hill, walk south for more great views from the Parkman Bandstand. Dedicated in 1912 and renovated in 1995, the bandstand still hosts concerts and performances.

- From the bandstand, walk south down the hill to the corner of Charles and Boylston streets and the Four Seasons Hotel, at 200 Boylston. Getting a cup of tea here, at the

Bristol Lounge, is a (relatively) cheap way to enjoy the opulence and grandeur of the Four Seasons without having to pony up for a room.

● From the hotel, either reenter the park for a final stroll down the canopied path toward the gate at the Arlington St. entrance or continue down bustling Boylston to your starting point at the Arlington T Station.

POINTS OF INTEREST

Swan Boats Public Garden Lagoon, Boston, MA 02108, 617-522-1966
Boston Common visitors center 147 Tremont St., Boston, MA 02108, 617-536-4100
Frog Pond Boston Common, Boston, MA 02108, 617-635-2120
Four Seasons Hotel 200 Boylston St., Boston, MA 02116, 617-338-4400

ROUTE SUMMARY

1. Begin at the Arlington T Station and enter the Public Garden at the corner of Arlington and Boylston streets.
2. Bear right and walk around the east side of the lagoon to the swan boats.
3. Continue to the northeast corner of the garden to the *Make Way for Ducklings* statues.
4. Head southwest along the north side of the lagoon to the gates at the corner of Commonwealth Ave. and Arlington St.
5. From the gates, walk east through the garden to Charles St.
6. Cross Charles to enter Boston Common and turn right on the path following Charles St. to the Central Burying Ground.
7. From the burying ground, turn left on the straight path heading northeast to the visitors center.
8. Walk behind the visitors center and take the center of the three paths to head northwest, past the Great Elm to Frog Pond.
9. From Frog Pond, turn left and head west to the Soldiers and Sailors Monument.
10. From the monument, walk south to the Parkman Bandstand.
11. From the bandstand, walk south down the hill to the corner of Boylston and Charles streets.
12. Turn right on Boylston to return to the Arlington T Station.

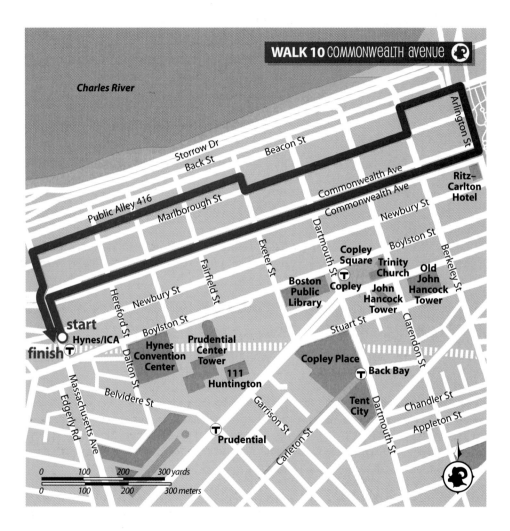

Charles River

Storrow Dr
Back St
Beacon St

Public Alley 416
Marlborough St

Commonwealth Ave
Commonwealth Ave

Ritz–
Carlton
Hotel

Arlington St

Newbury St

Exeter St
Dartmouth St
Boylston St

Berkeley St

Fairfield St
Copley Square
Trinity Church
Old John Hancock Tower

Hereford St
Newbury St
Boston Public Library
Copley
John Hancock Tower

start
Hynes/ICA
finish

Boylston St
Stuart St
Clarendon St

Dalton St
Hynes Convention Center
Prudential Center Tower
Copley Place
Back Bay

111 Huntington

Massachusetts Ave
Edgerly Rd
Belvidere St
Garrison St
Tent City
Dartmouth St
Chandler St
Appleton St

Carleton St
Prudential

0   100   200   300 yards
0   100   200   300 meters

10 COMMONWEALTH avenue: statues and saucer magnolias

BOUNDARIES: Commonwealth Ave., Arlington St., Beacon St., Massachusetts Ave.
DISTANCE: Approx. 2 miles
DIFFICULTY: Easy
PARKING: There is parking at the Prudential Center Parking Garage, accessed from Dalton St., Belvidere St., Exeter St., and Huntington Ave.
PUBLIC TRANSIT: Hynes Convention Center T Station; busses 1, CT1, and 55

The long, wide avenues of Boston's Back Bay are no accident. Built on mud flats, the neighborhood was designed as a showcase for Boston's wealth, with Commonwealth Ave. the proud centerpiece. From the Eliot Hotel at one end, to the statue of George Washington at the other, Commonwealth is the grand face that Victorian Boston built to display its wealth and respectability to the world. It is also the crucial link in the Emerald Necklace series of parks running from Jamaica Plain to the Boston Common.

There is no better time for this walk than on a bright, spring Sunday morning either before or after brunch. On those days, there are multitudes of families and young lovers out enjoying a stroll with the joy and relief that comes after a New England winter. It's also the perfect time to see the saucer magnolias planted at the behest of longtime Back Bay resident Laura Dwight along Commonwealth Ave.

● Begin at the very start of the Commonwealth Ave. pedestrian mall, at the intersection of Commonwealth and Massachusetts avenues. From here, it's possible to see the procession of statues and monuments that line Commonwealth. Along each side of Commonwealth are rows of houses ranging from ornate Italianate designs to clean, Federalist brick styles.

Begin your march down the center of the mall, heading east toward the Public Garden. The mall, designed by Arthur Gilman in 1856, features an array of gorgeous elms, sweet gum, maple, ash, and linden. It also boasts a veritable parade of honorable men (and three women) from Boston's past: Alexander Hamilton, Revolutionary

War soldier John Glover, former Boston mayor Patrick Collins, abolitionist William Lloyd Garrison, as well as a few more obscure individuals, including historian Samuel Morison, Argentinean president Domingo Sarmiento, and the explorer Leif Eriksson.

● After crossing Gloucester St., stop for a moment beside the one monument on the boulevard that celebrates all that women have achieved in and contributed to Boston. The Boston Women's Memorial, added in 2003 to commemorate Boston's rich women's heritage, features bronze statues of first lady and activist Abigail Adams, first-published African-American writer Phillis Wheatley, and journalist/suffragette Lucy Stone, along with excerpts from their written works etched upon the granite pedestals. The simplicity of the layout, along with descriptions of what these women achieved, make it one of the more moving installations on Commonwealth. It is also one of only a few sculptures in the city designed by a woman, in this case Meredith Gang Bergmann.

● Cross Dartmouth St. to see a powerful but somber black sculpture. The Vendome Hotel Memorial is dedicated to the nine firefighters who lost their lives in the Vendome Hotel Fire on June 17, 1972. Created in 1997 by

BACK STORY: LAURA DWIGHT AND THE SAUCER MAGNOLIAS

The leaves of saucer magnolias are a dark pink at the base, blending to a snowy white near the tips. And Laura Dwight loved them. A longtime Back Bay resident and neighborhood activist in the 1960s, Dwight envisioned a solid row of saucer magnolias lining the brownstones of Commonwealth Ave.—a spring explosion of color to rival Washington D.C.'s Tidal Basin.

In 1963, Dwight, who was in her 60s at the time, joined the Neighborhood Association of the Back Bay and began working toward her idea. She knocked on resident's doors, asking them to support planting a magnolia in front of their house. For a small fee—$8 for a small tree and $20 for a much larger one—Dwight would arrange for delivery of the tree and provide the labor to plant it and care for it. By the fall of 1963, Dwight had recruited MIT students for help and commenced two successive seasons of plantings that resulted in a line of saucer magnolias down the sunny north side of Commonwealth, and another line of dogwoods along the shady south side.

Back Story: Filling Back Bay

Always a fan of large public works projects, Boston had, even before the Big Dig, a project that could have been called the "Big Fill." In 1814, the Boston and Roxbury Mill Corporation built a mill dam that cut off nearly 500 acres of tidal marsh in the mouth of the Charles River. Unfortunately, the area became horribly polluted, and by 1849, the city health department ruled that the area must be filled in. For that project, which began in September of 1857 and lasted until 1900, fill was brought in from the town of Needham to cover more than 450 acres with an average of 20 feet of dirt.

This wide expanse of new land quickly became one of Boston's most fashionable districts, and city planners were hoping to create a memorable layout emphasizing their city's new wealth following the North's victory in the Civil War. Looking to the French for inspiration, city planners modeled Commonwealth Ave.—a 240-foot-wide boulevard split down the middle with a 100-foot mall fringed by elms and dotted with statues—after French architect Georges Haussmann's wide Parisian streets.

Ted Clausen, the polished granite wall recalls Washington D.C.'s Vietnam Veteran's memorial. The brass detail of a fireman's jacket and gloves laid over the sculpture is touching, and the etched chronology of events and selected quotes from various firefighters tells a story of heroism and tragedy.

● Continue down the center of the mall, passing Claremont and Berkeley streets before reaching Arlington St. (If you haven't caught the trick to the streets yet, notice that they are in alphabetical order.) The orderly procession of streets emphasizes the orderliness of the area, which contrasts with the jumble of streets and intersection that defines much of the city.

● As you near the Public Garden, you'll notice a figure seated on a horse beginning to rise above Arlington St. This is George Washington, 38 feet tall, leading the charge up Commonwealth. The statue was completed in 1869 by Charlestown sculptor Thomas Ball, who is also noted for having taught Daniel Chester French, the artist who created the Lincoln Memorial, Concord's Minuteman, and the statue of John Harvard. The George Washington statue is a grand entrance to the formal walkways of the Public Garden.

- Turn left on Arlington St. and continue to Beacon St.

- Turn left on Beacon St. and follow it to the Gibson House Museum at 137 Beacon. This brownstone and red brick Victorian mansion was built in 1860 and was occupied by the widow Catherine Hammond Gibson and her son, Charles. The Italian Renaissance townhouse features black walnut woodwork, imported carpets, and much of the Gibson family's furniture. Its afternoon tours (Wednesday through Sunday) offer glimpses into a pristine, if dark, Victorian household.

- Continue west on Beacon to Berkeley St., and turn left. Walk two blocks to the intersection of Berkeley St. and Marlborough St. On the corner, note the First and Second Church of Boston. Originally built in 1867, much of the church burned down in 1968. The ensuing renovation did a wonderful job of blending the old and new, right down to the striations in the brick.

- At Marlborough St., turn right and walk to 53 Marlborough, where you can get your Francophile fix at the French Library and Cultural Center. The building has a cozy library and often screens French films in the evenings.

- Turn right on Exeter St. and follow it to Public Alley 416.

- Turn left on Public Alley 416 and follow it up to Massachusetts Ave. This alley (and the many like it throughout Boston) offers an intimate glimpse of the casual backs of the brownstones that face the street. There are secret porches and patios that give a taste of their residents' real lives. Please also note that the residents use the alleyways to access their parking spaces, so beware of cars zipping down these alleys.

- At Massachusetts Ave., turn left to return to your starting point.

POINTS OF INTEREST

Gibson House Museum 137 Beacon St., Boston, MA 02116, 617-267-6338
First and Second Church of Boston 66 Marlborough St., Boston, MA 02116, 617-267-6730
French Library and Cultural Center 53 Marlborough St., Boston, MA 02116, 617-912-0400

route summary

1. Begin at the very start of the Commonwealth Ave. pedestrian mall, at the intersection of Commonwealth and Massachusetts avenues, and head northeast down the center of the promenade.
2. Turn left on Arlington St.
3. Turn left on Beacon St.
4. Turn left on Berkeley St.
5. Turn right on Marlborough St.
6 Turn right on Exeter St.
7. Turn left on Public Alley 416.
8. Turn left on Massachusetts Ave. to return to your starting point.

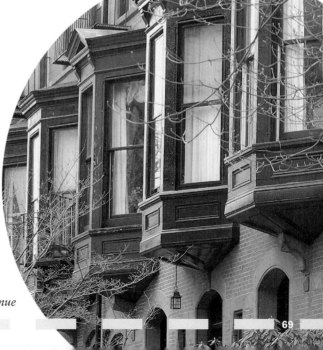

Oriel windows along Commonwealth Avenue

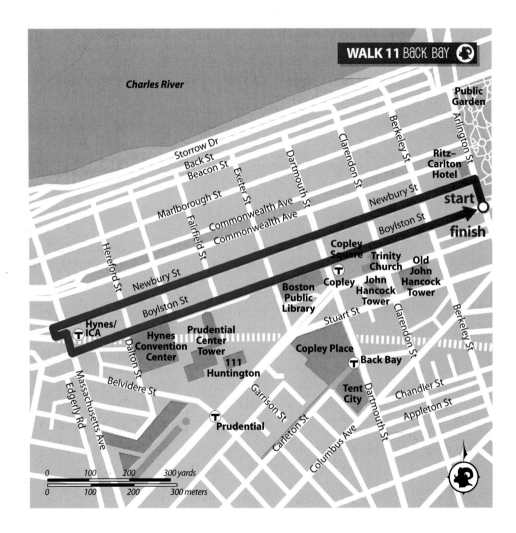

Charles River

Storrow Dr
Back St
Beacon St
Marlborough St
Commonwealth Ave
Commonwealth Ave
Newbury St
Boylston St
Newbury St
Boylston St

Exeter St
Fairfield St
Hereford St

Dartmouth St
Clarendon St
Berkeley St
Arlington St

Public
Garden

Ritz–
Carlton
Hotel

start

finish

Copley
Square
Copley

Trinity
Church
John
Hancock
Tower

Old
John
Hancock
Tower

Boston
Public
Library

Hynes/
ICA

Stuart St

Hynes
Convention
Center

Prudential
Center
Tower

111
Huntington

Dalton St
Belvidere St
Massachusetts Ave
Edgerly Rd

Prudential

Garrison St
Carleton St

Copley Place

Back Bay

Tent
City

Columbus Ave
Dartmouth St
Clarendon St
Berkeley St

Chandler St
Appleton St

0   100   200   300 yards
0   100   200   300 meters

11 Back Bay: and to think I found it on Newbury street

BOUNDARIES: **Newbury St., Massachusetts Ave., Boylston St., Arlington St.**
DISTANCE: **Approx. 2 miles**
DIFFICULTY: **Easy**
PARKING: **Boston Common Parking Garage on Charles St.**
PUBLIC TRANSIT: **Arlington T Station on the Green Line; busses 9, 10, 39, and 55**

Home to numerous trendy boutiques and upscale shops, this buyer's boulevard is well stocked with art, fashion, and food. Just be sure to bring all your spare change—and maybe a piece of plastic or two.

During the summer, the sidewalks fill with strolling shoppers and sightseers, creating a lively and pleasant atmosphere. If it gets too hot, duck into one of the stores or galleries to cool off. Or wait until the halfway point of this walk and treat yourself to something cold and sweet at one of the Boston ice cream institutions, J.P. Licks. Although this walk is mapped as an up-and-down straight walk, your path may be somewhat less linear. There are plenty of attractions to tempt you from the straight and narrow.

● Begin at the Arlington Street Church, at 351 Boylston (the corner of Arlington and Boylston streets). Before going down Newbury, duck inside to check out this soaring and impressive sanctuary. Designed by Arthur Gilman (who also designed the layout of Back Bay) and completed in 1861, it is the oldest public building in Back Bay. Its present foundation rests on 999 wooden pilings driven into the watery mud of Back Bay. These pilings must remain submerged or they will rot. Also of note are the 11 Tiffany stained-glass windows lining the main hall and upper galleries. This is believed to be the largest collection of Tiffany windows in a single church.

After you emerge from the cool darkness of the church, let your eyes adjust to the light, and then walk northwest toward Newbury St.

● Turn left on Newbury St. and head west. At 15 Newbury St. (on the right) is the prestigious Emmanuel Church. Also built in 1861, the church is famous for its lovely main sanctuary and Leslie Lindsey Memorial Chapel, as well as the Bach cantatas performed each Sunday during the 10 AM service. Continue west on Newbury St.

Stop at the double wooden doors of the New England Historic Genealogical Society, at 101 Newbury, to get in touch with your roots. Just inside the cool foyer are a small bookstore and a library, where, for $15, you can spend the day hunting down your family history or simply enjoying this quiet bit of Newbury. (There are bathrooms here.)

Continue down Newbury St., where the churches and art galleries begin to give way to clothing stores. Purveyors of clothing have stiff competition here, and many of the shops might not even outlast the clothing they sell. However, there are a few stand-outs that define Newbury St.—for example, Louis Boston, located at 234 Berkeley St., in a grand, red brick French-American building on the southwest corner of Newbury and Berkeley. Louis Boston is one of the city's more prestigious addresses for fine threads and housewares for the rich and occasionally famous. There is also a restaurant on the premises, but what is most interesting is the building itself. Constructed in 1863 by William Preston, it was the home of the Boston Society of Natural History before it moved in 1947 and became the Museum of Science.

From the rarefied air of Louis Boston, return to Newbury St. and turn left. For the more sporty, there is Niketown (200 Newbury) and Life is Good (283 Newbury). Niketown's 9,000 square feet of swooshness and outrageous prices make it a spectacle for tourists from around the world. Meanwhile, at Life is Good, you can find locally designed clothes and accessories that feature the happy stick figure known as Jake doing everything from playing a guitar to kayaking.

For the sweeter side of Newbury, it's a toss-up between the moose with a conscience (Emack & Bolio's, at 290 Newbury) or the powerhouse heifer from Jamaica Plain (J.P. Licks, at 352 Newbury). You can't go wrong—both shops offer locally made ice cream with fresh ingredients and interesting flavor combinations.

Newbury Comics (at 332 Newbury) is actually a great place to browse the latest CDs, DVDs, and eclectic toys (Scooby Doo lunchboxes anyone?), but not that many comic books. Trident Booksellers and Cafe (at 338 Newbury) is the place to go for more high-brow entertainment. With comfy chairs and a cafe, this is a perfect location to lounge over a cappuccino and a book.

If all this shopping has done you in, cross Massachusetts Ave. to the Other Side Cosmic Cafe, at 407 Newbury, for a cold beer with a decidedly anti-mercantile crowd. When the weather is nice, snag a table outside and watch the hordes of Berklee College of Music students and tourists tromp down Massachusetts Ave.

● From the Other Side, retrace your steps to Massachusetts Ave. and turn right to head one block south.

● Turn left on Boylston St. After one block, you come to the Boylston Street Fire Station at 941 Boylston. Still the home of Engine Company 33 and Ladder Company 15, this was the first combined fire and police station in the city when it opened in 1887. Take note of its remarkable Richardsonian Romanesque-style turret (used for drying hoses) and its handsome brick edifice. The fire station is such an architectural gem that when new equipment required wider doors, they decided to modify the equipment rather than change the façade. For more information, stop and chat with the firemen who often sit outside. They are very friendly and particularly good with kids.

Continue down Boylston for more shopping, with a slight difference. While Newbury St. has managed to attract and retain a number of local merchants, Boylston St. is more about household stores with household names. Get started with Crate and Barrel at 777 Boylston, then move on to stock the wine cellar at Best Cellars (745 Boylston). More knickknacks are available at Restoration Hardware, at 711 Boylston.

As you venture past the Boston Public Library (700 Boylston), you may feel the urge to run. There's a reason for that: This is the finish line of the famed Boston Marathon, which takes place annually on the third Monday in April, on Patriot's Day. Look for the finish line of the 26.2-mile race painted right on Boylston St. just before the intersection with Dartmouth Ave. Traffic is often heavy here, so don't practice your marathon form by sprinting down the center of the street.

Instead, continue down Boylston to the Beaux Arts masterpiece Berkeley Building, at 420 Boylston. Built in 1906 and renovated in 1989, this steel and glass structure is a registered Boston landmark and houses a number of offices. It's worth ducking inside for a look at the six-story atrium.

● Cross to the north side of Boylston and continue east for one of the best places in town for a sandwich, the Parish Cafe (361 Boylston). Many of Boston's top chefs have created unique sandwiches expressly for the Parish Cafe, and you'll find unusual combinations like banana nut bread with smoked ham and mango chutney or teriyaki tuna with wasabi on scallion focaccia. The Parish Cafe is also a great nightspot; it's one of the city's few places that serves food until 1 AM, with a last call for alcohol at 2 AM.

End at your starting point, at the Arlington Street Church.

POINTS OF INTEREST

Arlington Street Church 351 Boylston St., Boston, MA 02116, 617-536-7050

Emmanuel Church 15 Newbury St., Boston, MA 02116, 617-536-3355

New England Historic Genealogical Society 101 Newbury St., Boston, MA 02116, 617-536-5740

Louis Boston 234 Berkeley St., Boston, MA 02116, 800-225-5135

Niketown 200 Newbury St., Boston, MA 02116, 617-267-3400

Life is Good 283 Newbury St., Boston, MA 02116, 617-867-8900

Emack & Bolio's 290 Newbury St., Boston, MA 02115, 617-536-7127

J.P. Licks 352 Newbury St., Boston, MA 02115, 617-236-1666

Newbury Comics 332 Newbury St., Boston, MA 02115, 617-236-4930

Trident Booksellers and Cafe 338 Newbury St., Boston, MA 02115, 617-267-8688

Other Side Cosmic Cafe 407 Newbury St., Boston, MA 02115, 617-536-8437

Crate and Barrel 777 Boylston St., Boston, MA 02116, 617-262-8700

Best Cellars 745 Boylston St., Boston, MA 02116, 617-266-2900

Restoration Hardware 711 Boylston St., Boston, MA 02116, 617-578-0088

Boston Public Central Library 700 Boylston St., Boston, MA 02116, 617-536-5400

Parish Cafe 361 Boylston St., Boston, MA 02116, 617-247-4777

route summary

1. Start at the Arlington Street Church, at the corner of Arlington and Boylston streets, and follow Arlington north to Newbury St.

2. Turn left on Newbury and walk to the Other Side Cosmic Cafe, at 407 Newbury St.

3. Retrace your steps to Massachusetts Ave. and turn right.

4. Turn left on Boylston St. and follow it to your starting point at the corner of Arlington St.

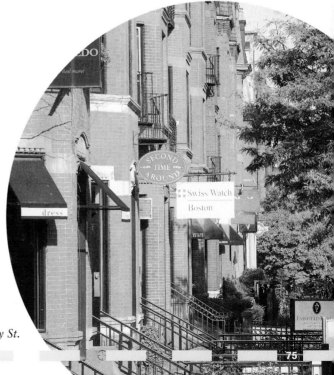

Shops along Newbury St.

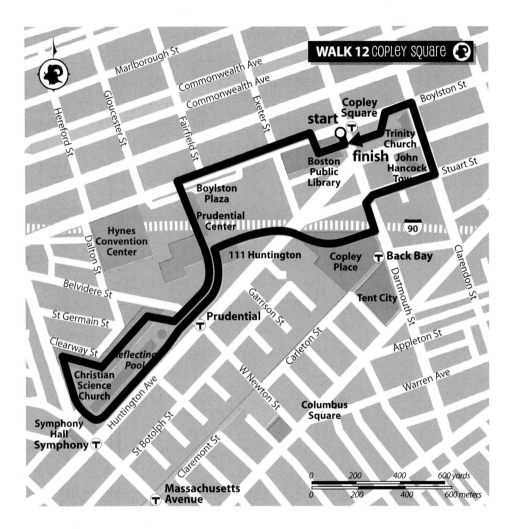

Marlborough St

Commonwealth Ave

Commonwealth Ave

Boylston St

Copley Square

start

Trinity Church

finish

John Hancock Tower

Stuart St

Boston Public Library

Hereford St

Gloucester St

Fairfield St

Exeter St

Clarendon St

Boylston Plaza

Prudential Center

Hynes Convention Center

Dalton St

90

Belvidere St

111 Huntington

Copley Place

Back Bay

Dartmouth St

St Germain St

Prudential

Garrison St

Tent City

Appleton St

Clearway St

Reflecting Pool

Carleton St

Warren Ave

Christian Science Church

Huntington Ave

W Newton St

Columbus Square

Symphony Hall

Symphony

St Botolph St

Claremont St

Massachusetts Avenue

	200	400	600 yards
0	200	400	600 meters

12 COPLEY SQUARE: ROUNDING THE SQUARE

BOUNDARIES: **Boylston St., Clarendon St., Huntington Ave., Massachusetts Ave.**
DISTANCE: **2 miles**
DIFFICULTY: **Easy**
PARKING: **There is parking at the Prudential Center Parking Garage, accessed from Dalton St., Belvidere St., Exeter St., and Huntington Ave.**
PUBLIC TRANSIT: **Copley Square T Station on the Green Line; busses 9, 10, 39, 55, 500, 501, 504, 505, 553, 554, 556, and 558**

This tour begins with a library, meanders through malls, and swings through a domed sanctuary called the Mother Church. From a brass hare to a glass globe, there is plenty to take in, and given the number of shops, perhaps even more to take home.

The dark coolness of the library, the refreshing water of the fountains, and the air-conditioned stretches of malls make this a great antidote to the dog days of summer.

● From the Copley Square T Station, head south on Dartmouth St. to the Central Library of the Boston Public Library system. The formal symmetry of the Charles McKim-designed façade, the red tile of the roof and its green copper cresting, and the triple-arched main entrance make the Central Library one of Boston's most architecturally impressive buildings. And that's just the inside.

Walk through the main entrance into an impressive sanctuary of pink Knoxville and Levanto marble. As you climb the main staircase, listen for the tinkling of water just outside the windows. That's the only hint of the treasures to come. The building is just as fascinating as the broad-ranging collection of books it houses.

Continue up the stairs to the second floor, past the twin lions honoring Massachusetts Civil War infantry, and on to the hushed elegance of Bates Hall, with its barrel-arched ceilings and lines of brass lamps with green lantern shades. Art fans will want to check out the set of murals by famed Boston portraitist John Singer Sargent. To find these, continue up the main staircase to the third floor. Other attractions worth noting are the Puvis de Chavannes Gallery and the Abbey Room, with its series of murals by American artist Edwin Austin Abbey. Both are on the second floor. The third floor's Wiggin Gallery houses a collection of prints and drawings donated to the library.

Return to the first floor via the main staircase and turn left to find **Sebastian's Map Room Cafe**, with its vaulted ceiling and archival map theme. Get a cup of tea and head out to the Italianate courtyard by going around the corner and out the double doors. The water you heard earlier was from Frederick MacMonnies's *Bacchante and Infant Faun* in the courtyard of the Central Library. With high walls, a well-marked garden path, and the fountain, the courtyard is a lovely oasis. You can't even hear the sounds of the streets outside.

Leave through the courtyard doors opposite the ones you used to get here. This puts you in the Johnson Building, another library wing. Follow the signs to exit the library onto Boylston St.

● Turn left on Boylston and follow it to the Boylston Plaza on the left, just past the Mandarin Oriental Boston Hotel. The leaping, near-naked man in the center of the plaza is Donna De Lure's 5-ton bronze statue, *Quest Eternal*. This depiction of "humanity's noble pursuit of knowledge" seems an odd choice for the entrance to a mall—but perhaps this questing man also has more material pursuits. Ascend the staircase and cross the plaza to the entrance to the Prudential Center.

● Enter the Prudential Center through the large glass doors and walk through the food court, bearing left into the Boylston Arcade. This hall brings you to the Center Court and the South Courtyard. Transformed from what was once a dark, deserted, open-air strip mall, the Prudential Center has metamorphosed into a mall that any city would be proud to call its own. It feels light and airy—a marked contrast to Copley Place, which is all dark marble and brass. It also sits above the largest underground parking garage in New England—there are spaces for about 3,600 cars.

● From the Center Court, turn sharply right to the Prudential Arcade and the Prudential Tower. The 750-foot tower has 52 stories and was, for 15 years, the tallest building in Boston (the John Hancock Tower, featured later on this tour, scooped it). You can, of course, pay to go up to the Skywalk Observatory now, or make a note to come back here at sunset for a drink at the Top of the Hub restaurant.

- Either way, turn left to enter the Belvidere Arcade and head for the exit.

- Cross Belvidere St. and enter the Christian Science Church Park. At a large semicircle of hedges, bear right to walk along the northern edge of the reflecting pool. If the day is warm, you may find kids playing in the waters of the nearby fountain. The highlight of the Christian Science Church Park is the Mary Baker Eddy Library, with the Mapparium. Here, you can journey inside an enormous glass globe to get an entirely different perspective on the world as you know it—or at least as it was once was (the globe was mapped out in 1934). The library is open from 10 AM to 4 PM Tuesday through Sunday, and the final tour of the Mapparium is available at 3:30 PM.

  To get there, bear right around the domed sanctuary known as the "Mother Church" (it's the headquarters of the First Church of Christ, Scientist) on the southwestern corner of the Christian Science Church Park and head to the main entrance of the library at the western edge of the park (along Massachusetts Ave.).

- Exit the park on Huntington Ave. and turn left.

- Reenter the Prudential Center through the Huntington entrance. Continue down the Huntington Arcade to the Winter Garden.

- Turn right at the Back Bay Arcade, and follow it to Bridge Court and the Copley Bridge.

- Take the Copley Bridge to Copley Place, a more upscale mall, with stores like Coach and Christian Dior. Continue straight through the central hall, and take a left at the Neiman Marcus to exit at Stuart St.

Fountain in Boston Public Library courtyard

- Turn right to head east on Stuart St. to Clarendon St.

- Turn left on Clarendon and follow it to Copley Square. At 200 Clarendon is the John Hancock Tower. Designed by Henry Cobb of I.M. Pei's architecture firm, this glass-lined tower is 790 feet tall, with 60 floors. It is the tallest building in Boston and certainly one of the most recognizable—which is not always a good thing. It has been a target of controversy since day one, garnering outrage for foundation collapses, glass panes falling to the ground below, and other structural deficiencies. When many of the missing windows were replaced with plywood, the building was dubbed the "Plywood Palace." These defects have all been fixed, however, and the tower now provides a great photo opportunity for shutterbugs who like to contrast the tan stone of nearby Trinity Church with the 10,344 modern glass panels of the Hancock Tower.

- Enter Copley Square from the corner of Clarendon and Boylston streets. You are standing on the north side of Trinity Church, at 206 Clarendon, which anchors one end of Copley Square. Trinity Church was finished in 1877, and despite its mélange of architectural styles, it fits in well with the grand façade of the Boston Public Library (on the opposite side of Copley Square) and the Copley Plaza Hotel. Stop inside to see the stained-glass windows of this famed H.H. Richardson sanctuary.

   In the center of Copley Square, near the fountain, are two bronze creatures, the *Tortoise and Hare* sculptures, which celebrate the finish line of the Boston Marathon.

   If you happen to be walking on a Tuesday or Friday, snoop around the Copley Square Farmer's Market. Dozens of vendors proffer locally grown produce and flowers, handcrafted gifts, and assorted organic munchies.

- Cross to the western side of Copley Square to return to the Copley Square T Station.

POINTS OF INTEREST

Boston Public Central Library 700 Boylston St., Boston, MA 02116, 617-536-5400

Prudential Center 800 Boylston St., Boston, MA 02199, 617-236-3100

Mary Baker Eddy Library 200 Massachusetts Ave., Boston, MA 02115, 888-222-3711

Copley Place 2 Copley Pl., Boston, MA 02116, 617-369-5000

John Hancock Tower 200 Clarendon St., Boston, MA 02116, 617-572-6000

Copley Square Farmer's Market Copley Square along St. James Ave., Boston, MA 02116, Tuesdays and Fridays, 11 AM to 6 PM

route summary

1. From the Copley Square T Station, head south on Dartmouth St. to the Boston Public Library.
2. Enter the library through the front gates.
3. Exit the library via the Johnson Building and turn left on Boylston St.
4. Follow Boylston to Boylston Plaza, on the left, and ascend the stairs to the North Terrace.
5. Enter the Prudential Center through the glass food court doors.
6. Exit the Prudential Center via the Belvidere Arcade.
7. Cross Belvidere St. to enter the Christian Science Church Park.
8. Walk counterclockwise through the park and exit on Huntington Ave. by turning left on Huntington.
9. Reenter the Prudential Center at the Huntington entrance and cross to Copley Place via the Copley Bridge.
10. Exit Copley Place by the doors near Neiman Marcus and turn right on Stuart St. to head east.
11. Turn left on Clarendon St.
12. Enter Copley Square from the corner of Clarendon and Boylston streets.
13. Cross to the western side of Copley Square to return to the Copley Square T Station.

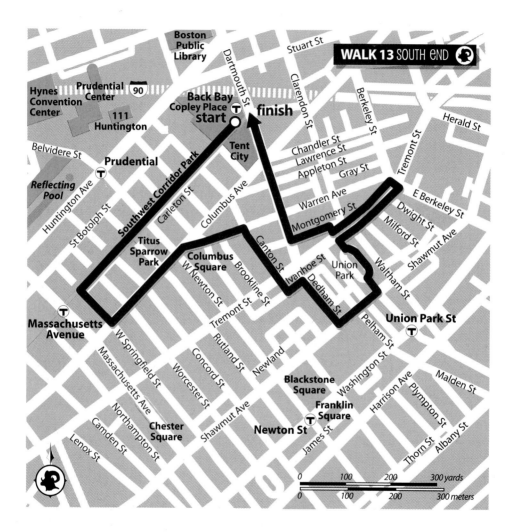

13 SOUTH END: Green Spaces, Local Activism, and a Cyclorama

BOUNDARIES: Copley Pl., Massachusetts Ave., Shawmut Ave., Berkeley St.
DISTANCE: Approx. 2½ miles
DIFFICULTY: Easy
PARKING: A limited amount of free, two-hour parking is available along Columbus Ave. and Dartmouth St.
PUBLIC TRANSIT: Back Bay T Station; busses 9, 10, and 43

Green spaces, historic brownstones, modern steel and glass, good cheap food, great expensive food—this route includes much of what makes Boston the perfect walking town. Beginning at the Back Bay T station, this walk tours the city's largest historic district—a 500-acre area featuring everything from contemporary literature, inspirational stories, and New England's largest collection of Victorian brownstone townhouses.

Although this walk is still charming in the dark of winter, it is best in the spring when the community gardens and flower boxes are in full bloom.

● **Start on the west side of Dartmouth St. in the Dartmouth Courtyard (directly across the street from the Back Bay T Station). Before setting off, take a moment to read Jane Barnes's short story "Counterpoint," and Ruth Whitman's poem "If My Boundary Stops Here," which are etched into the granite pillars set into the middle of the brick plaza. They are just two of the 18 literary works from local writers inscribed at various places throughout the Southwest Corridor Park, a 4.7-mile, 50-acre greenway stretching from the Back Bay T Station to Jamaica Plain. The Southwest Corridor Park was developed in the 1980s after local citizens fought a proposed 12-lane highway running from Cambridge to Route 128.**

Also note the building at 130 Dartmouth St. called "Tent City." On April 27, 1968, activists, fed up with the urban renewal programs that had been demolishing low-income housing for things like parking garages and office buildings, gathered in a parking lot that stood on what had been houses and was destined to become a parking garage.

As their numbers swelled to 400, the protestors put up tents and wooden shanties, played music, grilled hamburgers, and invited the media to cover the event. Along with the television cameras, thousands of people arrived, and a festive atmosphere ensued. After four days, the protesters decamped and created the Tent City Task Force, which eventually became the Tent City Corporation. Exactly 20 years after the protest, the Tent City Apartments were constructed, providing mixed-income housing—with a parking garage *below* the housing complex.

● From Tent City, follow the Southwest Corridor Park southwest roughly a third of a mile down to Claremont Park. As you walk, you can make stops at the Carlton Dog Park and playground, or shoot hoops at the basketball court on the left in Rutland Square.

● Turn left on Claremont Park, which is not really a park at all but a lovely residential street leading to Columbus Ave. Traipse down the crooked brick sidewalk (watch your step!) to 5 Claremont Park to check out the tree growing up the side of the building. Also note the lovely doors and bay windows along this section.

● At the corner of Claremont Park and Columbus Ave. is the Columbus Cafe and Bar (at 535 Columbus Ave.), a great place to nip in for a coffee and pastry. Or get a more substantial meal at the House of Siam (542 Columbus Ave.), just across Columbus Ave.

● Turn left on Columbus Ave. If you can wait to eat, journey northeast to the Cafe Amsterdam, at 517 Columbus, and treat yourself to a grilled panini.

● Take your sandwich one block down to Columbus Square and eat it in Harriet Tubman Park, on the other side of Columbus Ave., with the two monuments to Boston's black heritage. The 10-foot-tall bronze statue, *Step on Board*, features abolitionist and Underground Railroad leader Harriet Tubman bringing slaves to freedom. Created in 1999, it was the first statue on city-owned land honoring a woman (there are a few more now). The other monument in the square honors the Emancipation Proclamation and was done in 1913 by black artist Meta Warner Fuller.

- After your rest, head northeast on Warren Ave. The round building of the Concord Baptist Church, at 190 Warren, will be on your right. This dignified church with a circular tower was where a young Martin Luther King, Jr., cut his ministerial teeth while studying theology at Boston University.

- Turn right on Canton St., where you pass another lovely playground on the corner.

- Follow Canton until it bends sharply to the right and becomes Aguadilla St. Here, follow the sidewalk that leads directly to the tile mural dedicated to Ramón Emeterio Bantances, a physician who worked to save Puerto Ricans from cholera while actively trying to abolish slavery. The brightly colored tile mural includes other, more local Puerto Rican heroes like the ones in the 1960s who helped create Villa Victoria, an affordable housing complex that was once slated to be replaced with luxury apartments.

- Cross the square to W. Dedham St., and turn right.

- Turn left on Shawmut Ave. If you haven't been tempted to grab a bite yet, walk to the South End Buttery, at 314 Shawmut. You may want to try one of the three types of cupcakes named after the owners' dogs.

- Turn left on Union Park for another ramble through a quiet, tree-lined neighborhood street. Some claim that Union Park rivals Beacon Hill's Louisburg Square; certainly, when spring brings out flowers like black-eyed Susans, the contrast with the surrounding brick houses is stunning. You be the judge.

Harriet Tubman Park

- Turn right on Tremont St. and follow it to the Berkeley Community Gardens at Public Alley 705. In the springtime, these gardens burst with vegetables and flowers. The land is owned by the South End/Lower Roxbury Open Space Land Trust, which rents plots for a yearly fee.

- From the gardens, cross Tremont and turn around to walk back on Tremont on the opposite side of the street to enjoy urban renewal at its best. First, stop by Sibling Rivalry, a restaurant with an intriguing concept. Two brothers, both chefs, offer a menu featuring the creations of one brother on one side and the other brother's offerings on the opposite side.

The Boston Center for the Arts (BCA) is located in the set of buildings starting at 539 Tremont St. with the Calderwood Theater. This nonprofit visual and performing arts complex consists of four theaters, the Mills Gallery, the Artists Studio Building, the Boston Ballet Building, and the Community Music Center of Boston. However, the most intriguing space in the BCA complex is the Cyclorama Building, at 541 Tremont. The Cyclorama was built in 1884 to house massive, 365-degree paintings known as cycloramas. The first cyclorama was painted by Parisian Paul Dominique Philippoteaux and featured a rendition of the Battle of Gettysburg. Viewers came in through a long hallway and walked up a staircase so they were completely surrounded by the painting, which was 50 feet high and 400 feet long. Actual guns, bushes, sandbags, and statues of soldiers placed in the center of the painting gave viewers the impression they were right in the action. Once the popularity of this type of art died down, the building served a range of purposes, including a roller-skating rink, boxing ring, flower exchange, and factory before its current incarnation as a performance hall for the BCA.

Next door to the Cyclorama is Tremont Estates, which houses studio and rehearsal spaces, the Mills Gallery, and the Boston Ballet Building. Nestled in the bottom, Tremont Estates is one of Boston's best restaurants, Hamersley's Bistro, a bright and cheerful French restaurant. It's the perfect place for dinner before a show at the BCA.

If the menu there doesn't entice, cross to the eastern side of Tremont and try B & G Oysters. This tiny seafood bistro, done up in cool blue tiles and polished steel, is dominated by a long counter with a dozen or so seats, where you can watch the chefs in action. Alternatively, snag a table in the delightful back patio for a "hidden garden" experience.

If you are in the mood for something a bit less fishy, cross Waltham St. to 552 Tremont St. for the Butcher Shop. This small restaurant and gourmet butchery is for the meat lover, but it also is a popular night spot.

- From the corner of Waltham St. and Tremont, continue west for one block and turn right on Union Park for a quick jog to Montgomery St.

- Turn left on Montgomery and follow it to Dartmouth St.

- At Dartmouth, turn right and stop at the Haley House Corner Shop, at 23 Dartmouth St. Haley House began as a soup kitchen in 1966, and in 1996, after 30 years of serving hot meals to the city's homeless people, it began training its guests in baking. Those who went through the job training were then able to sell their goodies to the people in the neighborhood, who were attracted by the aroma of their fresh-baked treats. Building off this success, Haley House opened a cafe in Roxbury in 2003 and now the much-expanded job training program is housed there. The corner shop on Dartmouth, which sells the cafe's baked goods, supports the Roxbury social enterprise and job-training program. Stop here for one of their homemade baked goods or a cup of delicious soup—all made by individuals on the road to economic independence.

- Continue north on Dartmouth St. to your starting point at the Dartmouth Courtyard.

POINTS OF INTEREST

Columbus Cafe and Bar 535 Columbus Ave., Boston, MA 02118, 617-247-9001

House of Siam 542 Columbus Ave., Boston, MA 02118, 617-267-1755

Cafe Amsterdam 517 Columbus Ave., Boston, MA 02118, 617-437-6400

Harriet Tubman Park Columbus Ave. and Warren St., Boston, MA 02118, 617-266-0022

Concord Baptist Church 190 Warren Ave., Boston, MA 02118, 617-266-8062

South End Buttery 314 Shawmut Ave., Boston, MA 02118, 617-482-1015

Sibling Rivalry 525 Tremont St., Boston, MA 02118, 617-338-5338

Boston Center for the Arts 539 Tremont St., Boston, MA 02118, 617-426-5000

Hamersley's Bistro 553 Tremont St., Boston, MA 02118, 617-423-2700

B & G Oysters 550 Tremont St., Boston, MA 02118, 617-423-0550

Butcher Shop 552 Tremont St., Boston, MA 02118, 617-423-4800

Haley House Corner Shop 23 Dartmouth St., Boston, MA 02118, 617-236-8132

route summary

1. Begin at the Dartmouth Courtyard across the street from the Back Bay T Station and follow the Southwest Corridor Park southwest.

2. Turn left on Claremont Park.

3. Turn left on Columbus Ave.

4. Bear right on Warren Ave.

5. Turn right on Canton St.

6. Walk through Villa Victoria to W. Dedham St. and turn right.

7. Turn left on Shawmut Ave. and walk to South End Buttery at 314 Shawmut.

8. Retrace your steps on Shawmut and turn right on Union Park.

9. Turn right on Tremont St. and follow it to Berkeley St.

10. Retrace your steps on the other side of Tremont St. and turn right on Union Park.

11. Turn right on Montgomery St.

12. Turn right on Dartmouth St. to return to your starting point.

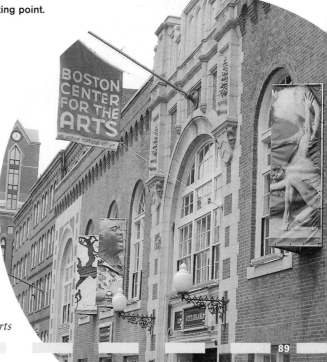

Boston Center for the Arts

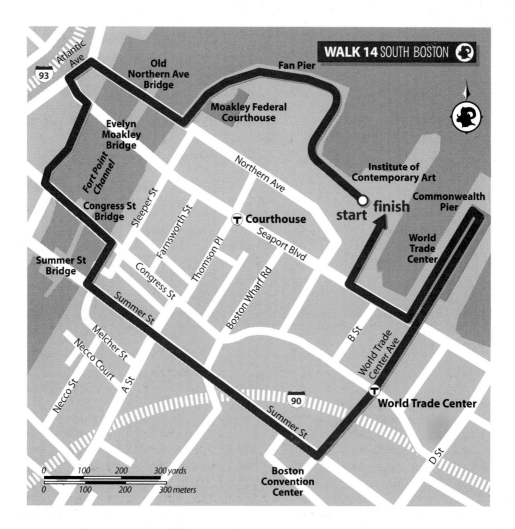

14 SOUTH BOSTON: COMMERCE, HIGH ART, LAW, AND A REALLY BIG MILK BOTTLE

BOUNDARIES: **Northern Ave., Atlantic Ave., and Summer St., World Trade Center Ave.**
DISTANCE: **Approx 2½ miles**
DIFFICULTY: **Easy**
PARKING: **Paid parking is available on Congress St. and Northern Ave.**
PUBLIC TRANSIT: **World Trade Center on the Silver Line (actually a bus with a free transfer from the Red Line); busses 4 and 7**

Start near the water between Anthony's Pier 4 restaurant and the Institute of Contemporary Art. To your right is a Boston institution, the brick façade and old steam engine of Anthony's Pier 4, once the highest-grossing restaurant in the United States and one that has served U.S. presidents and celebrities alike. To the left are the stark lines and striking architecture of the Institute of Contemporary Art. Ahead is Boston Harbor, where massive tankers, slow-moving ferries, and recreational boats of all sorts navigate around each other. From here, this walk follows the paved path along the Fan Pier in front of the Moakley Federal Courthouse, across the Old Northern Ave. Bridge to the busy Atlantic Ave., back across the Fort Point Channel to the Children's Museum, and down to Summer St. for a lovely straight shot down to the Convention Center and World Trade Center.

I suggest a bright spring or fall day when the breezes are strong enough to clear the air for great views across the harbor to downtown and the mouth of the Mystic River. It's flat and safe enough for a stroller, with plenty for the kids to enjoy along the way.

● Beginning on the eastern side, Anthony's Pier 4 restaurant, at 140 Northern Ave., resist the urge for fried clams and creamy New England clam chowder and begin by walking east across the parking lot to the Institute of Contemporary Art (ICA). The ICA was once located in a smaller building on Back Bay's Boylston St., and it was moved to this home in the fall of 2006. Designed by Diller Scofidio + Renfro, the museum offers four floors and 65,000 shiny square feet of multimedia art installations, inter-active exhibits, and a cafe by Wolfgang Puck. Even a ride in the super-wide, glass-walled elevator is worth the $12 price of admission, but don't miss the Poss Family

Mediatheque, a steeply sloping auditorium dropped from the bottom of the building's cantilever. This uniquely designed room, which juts out from the building itself, features rows of computers hooked into art sites and links to the ICA independent films. The massive picture window at the bottom of the gallery is itself a work of art, offering a view focused entirely on the water, with neither sky nor horizon in view. As the architect herself envisioned, it is an ever-changing masterpiece.

If you're hungry, visit the Wolfgang Puck Water Cafe downstairs; otherwise, head outside to the Putnam Investments Plaza, a great place for relaxing and enjoying views of the water. The waterfront side of the plaza is part of Boston's 39-mile Harborwalk, which runs along the water throughout much of Boston.

- From ICA, head north along the Harborwalk, following the Fan Pier (named, of course, for its fan shape) in front of the Moakley Federal Courthouse. The path offers a view across the water at the glass façade of ICA, with the mediatheque hanging down like a dog's jaw. It then turns to reveal a lovely panorama of Boston Harbor and the waterfront.

- At the courthouse, stop to take in the various signs and exhibits about Boston's maritime heritage and the history of its waterfront. At the very top of the pier, take the paths on the left through the garden, with its plots of cinquefoil, fragrant sumac, roses, and summer sweet.

- Follow the path along the waterfront to the Old Northern Ave. Bridge. At the Barking Crab Restaurant, turn right onto Northern Ave. If you've already worked up an appetite, stop in for a lobster roll sandwich or the crab cakes. In the summer, the Barking Crab rocks out with live music on Tuesdays, Thursdays, and Sunday; in the winter, only Tuesdays are rockin'.

- Cross the pedestrian bridge to reach busy Atlantic Ave. This swinging truss bridge used to swivel in the middle to let boats through, but it is now solely for pedestrians.

- Turn left on Atlantic Ave. to head south. Before Boston's famed Big Dig, this part of Atlantic was dwarfed by overhead freeways. Now all that stuff is underground, and this section of the Financial District has a totally new face.

- Cross Seaport Blvd. at the Evelyn Moakley Bridge and immediately wind your way to the water behind Independence Wharf, at 470 Atlantic (look for the blue "Harborwalk" signs). The Independence Wharf building features a free, 14th-floor observation deck (open daily from 10 AM to 5 PM) and public, 24-hour restrooms.

- Head south along one of the newer Harborwalk sections through the open plaza, which has benches on the waterfront side of the glassy new Intercontinental Hotel (510 Atlantic Ave.).

  Continue south on the Harborwalk along Fort Point Channel as far as Congress St.

- Turn left on Congress to cross the Congress St. Bridge. Halfway across the bridge is the Boston Tea Party Ships and Museum, which will reopen in the summer of 2009. The new museum will feature 40,000 square feet of exhibits showing exactly what went down (besides a lot of tea!) that fateful December night in 1773. Particularly impressive will be the three replicas of the *Beaver,* the *Elinore*, and the *Dartmouth*—the three ships that were lightened of their loads.

- When you can't contain the kids (or your-self) any longer, continue over the bridge toward the giant milk bottle to the Children's Museum, at 300 Congress St. A massive renovation and expan-sion of the museum in 2007 included a glass and steel face that juts out from the brick of the old waterfront warehouse. If it weren't for the giant milk bottle in front and the PBS character Arthur sitting on the roof, the building might pass for a trendy computer software headquarters. But walk inside the front doors, where you encounter a three-story

Downtown Boston from South Boston's Fan Pier

climbing structure made from light, gleaming wood and rope nets—and it's obvious this place is for kids. If that doesn't make you wish you were a kid again, there are myriad other exhibitions that will, including a water area, basketball hoops, and a place where you can crawl underneath a cage with live turtles to get a worm's eye view of the reptiles. The secret is to show up at the Children's Museum just after 5 PM on Friday evenings, when admission is a mere dollar. The museum is, of course, open other hours (daily, from 10 AM to 5 PM, and Fridays until 9 PM), but admission is a bit steeper then ($10 for adults, $8 for kids).

● From the museum, walk over to the railing facing the Fort Point Channel. The shiny glass building is the Intercontinental Hotel you passed earlier. Facing the water, turn left and take the path along the water down to Summer St.

● Turn left on Summer to visit the Boston Wharf area, the center of the Boston wool trade for a century and a burgeoning artist community for the past 20 years. The Boston Wharf Company filled in the site from 1837 to 1882, using it first to store sugar and molasses and then mainly wool.

BacK STOrY: GOT (LOTS OF) MILK?

If the Hood milk bottle was real, it would hold 50,000 gallons of milk with 8,620 gallons of cream on the top. Unfortunately, the bottle is more than 70 years old, so it would also be a bit beyond the expiration date. The iconic structure was brought by boat to the Children's Museum in 1977 to serve snacks and drinks to museum-goers. Before that, it served ice cream along Route 44 in Taunton. Refurbished in 2007 along with the museum, the Hood milk bottle again dispenses snacks like hot dogs, ice cream, and, of course, Hood milk.

- At 274 Summer, stop at Marco Polo to gorge on huge servings of hot pasta, lovely homemade shepherd's pie, fresh sandwiches, or one of their specialty soups. Just down from Marco Polo, at 300 Summer, is the Fort Point Arts Connect Gallery, an exhibition space for local artists and members of Fort Point Arts Community, a nonprofit community organization founded in 1980.

- Continue along Summer, which becomes a raised road and eventually leads out of the tunnel of old warehouses-turned-office-buildings to an open space. To your left is a nice view of the Moakley Courthouse and the ICA. In front, rising like a massive ship on the horizon, is the Boston Convention and Exhibition Center. Boasting nearly a million square feet, this building anchors World Trade Center Ave. with the World Trade Center on the other side.

- Turn left on World Trade Center Ave. and walk toward the World Trade Center. Note the Andrei Pitynski statue, *The Partisans*, honoring the Polish and Jewish guerilla fighters from World War II. Walk through the stone archway past the offices, meeting spaces, hotels, and exhibition halls of Boston's World Trade Center. At the end of the center, you can step outside to the end of the Commonwealth Pier to access the Harborwalk, or just to enjoy the views of the harbor.

- Retrace your steps to the front of the World Trade Center near the parking lot and descend the stairs to rejoin Northern Ave. at water level. To the left is Fish Pier, which opened in 1914 and is the oldest continually working fish pier in the United States. You can see fishermen arriving with their catch from the end of the pier.

- Turn right on Northern Ave. to return to your starting point at Anthony's Pier 4 restaurant, where you can reward yourself with a meal of their famous seafood (try the scrod if it's fresh).

POINTS OF INTEREST

Anthony's Pier 4 140 Northern Ave., Boston, MA 02210, 617-482-6262

Institute of Contemporary Art 100 Northern Ave., Boston, MA 02210, 617-478-3101

Moakley Federal Courthouse 1 Courthouse Way, Boston, MA 02210, 617-261-2440

Barking Crab Restaurant 88 Sleeper St., Boston, MA 02210, 617-426-2722

Independence Wharf 470 Atlantic Ave., Boston, MA 02210, 617-273-8000

Intercontinental Hotel 510 Atlantic Ave., Boston, MA 02210, 617-747-1000

Boston Tea Party Ships and Museum Congress St. Bridge, Boston, MA 02210.
Note: This museum is closed for renovation until summer 2009.

Children's Museum 300 Congress St., Boston, MA 02210, 617-426-8855

Marco Polo 274 Summer St., Boston, MA 02210, 617-695-9039

Fort Point Arts Connect Gallery 300 Summer St., Boston, MA 02210, 617-423-4299

Boston Convention and Exhibition Center 415 Summer St., Boston, MA 02210, 617-954-2000

World Trade Center Boston 200 Seaport Blvd., Boston, MA 02210, 617-385-5000

ROUTE SUMMARY

1. Starting at Anthony's Pier 4 (140 Northern Ave.), follow Harborwalk north to the Old Northern Ave. Bridge.
2. Turn right on Northern Ave.
3. Turn left on Atlantic Ave.
4. Cross Seaport Blvd., and walk toward the water behind Independence Wharf.
5. Take the Harborwalk south along the Fort Point Channel.
6. Turn left on Congress St. and cross the Congress St. Bridge to the Children's Museum.
7. From the Children's Museum, follow the Harborwalk south.

8. Turn left on Summer St.

9. Turn left on World Trade Center Ave.

10. Walk through the World Trade Center to the end of Commonwealth Pier, and then retrace your steps to the front of the center.

11. Descend the stairs to water level.

12. Turn right on Northern Ave. to return to Anthony's Pier 4.

Fan Pier

1900

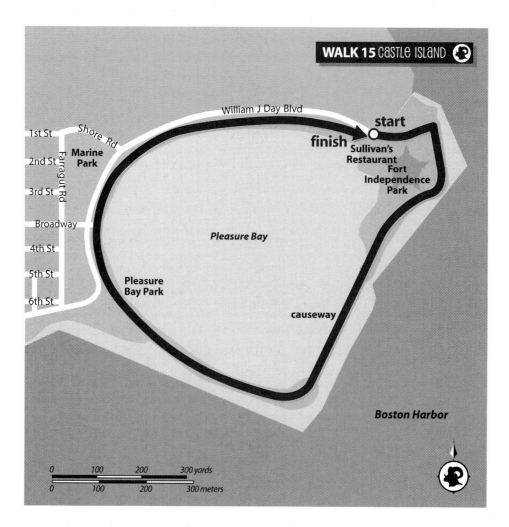

start

finish

William J Day Blvd

Shore Rd

1st St

2nd St

3rd St

Broadway

4th St

5th St

6th St

Farragut Rd

Marine Park

Sullivan's Restaurant

Fort Independence Park

Pleasure Bay

Pleasure Bay Park

causeway

Boston Harbor

0   100   200   300 yards

0   100   200   300 meters

15 Castle Island: From Independence to Pleasure and Back

BOUNDARIES: William J. Day Blvd.
DISTANCE: Approx. 2 miles
DIFFICULTY: Easy
PARKING: There is plenty of public parking along William J. Day Blvd. and near Fort Independence Park.
PUBLIC TRANSIT: JFK/UMass T Station on the Red Line; busses 9 and 11

Nestled against an industrial port, Castle Island and Pleasure Bay nonetheless offer miles of pleasant beach paths with views of sailboats and windsurfers. This walk starts at a historic fort and continues along a breakwater populated with people fishing for bass or just enjoying the view. The tour then loops back along the beach to the starting point—a terrific place for ice cream.

While it's great to be on the beach in the heat of summer, this area gets pretty crowded during those months. Instead, wait until everyone's gone back to school in early fall and pick a warm day to enjoy this stroll.

● Facing Fort Independence, take the path that leads to the left, in between Sullivan's Restaurant and the fort, to go around the fort clockwise. The pentagonal fort is the eighth edition of a fort on this site and was built between 1835 and 1851. (The first fort was constructed in 1644.) This 22-acre point of land was an island before it was connected with landfill (hence the name Castle Island) and occupies a strategic point guarding the entrance to the harbor. The British retreated here in the days after the Boston Massacre to ease the tensions downtown. On summer weekends, docents from the Department of Conservation and Recreation offer free, half-hour, guided tours from noon to 3:30 PM. If you decide to skip the tour in favor of some burgers and fries from Sullivan's, you can take your meal to the picnic tables inside the fort.

● About a quarter of the way around the fort, walk out on the pier on the left to watch the boat traffic in and out of Boston Harbor. But that's not the main attraction.

Situated just across a narrow spit of water from Boston's Logan Airport, you can watch 747s lumber down the runway and lift off just above your head. It's pretty impressive. Also keep an ear out for the (mostly) friendly verbal jousting among the bass fishermen who line the pier with their poles. It's a wonderful cacophony of dialects and diatribe.

- Continue to the eastern edge of the peninsula along the portion of the Harborwalk that leads around the fort, and walk out onto the breakwater path, heading south. From the breakwater, enjoy the views into Pleasure Bay and out to the harbor. This section is popular with walkers and joggers, so there is always plenty of activity along the walk. Where the path hits a roundabout and bears right to return to the mainland, take a moment to look out along the beach. You may catch windsurfers darting through the waters or kayakers paddling among the moored boats. Farther down the beach is the Curley Community Center, and beyond that is Carson Beach.

- Once back on land, turn right to walk along Pleasure Bay back to your starting point. This section of beach is popular with families whose young kids take advantage of the mild waves. If you'd

Back Story: The L Street Brownies

The L Street Brownies is a dedicated group of men, and since 1980, women who show up daily to take a swim in the waters in front of the Curley Community Center (also known as the L Street Bathhouse). Membership costs a dollar and ranges from 35 to 50 people at any given time. While they swim year-round, they are best known for their New Year's Day swim, an annual event that draws hundreds of swimmers, media, and spectators to the beach. Although residents have been swimming during the winter since the mid-19th century, the first documented New Year's Day swim was in 1904, when a reporter snapped a picture of it.

prefer to take a longer walk, you can extend this one by an additional 3 miles or so by turning left at the plaza and continuing along the boardwalk as far south as popular Carson Beach. Or, if you turn right, you can cross William J. Day Blvd. and wander through the various athletic fields of Marine Park.

Once you've returned to the starting point, reward yourself with something from Sullivan's. Like many beachside burger joints, it has no inside seating and is not open during the winter. It does have a loyal following, though, and you'll hear plenty of South Boston accents and probably a few Irish brogues.

POINTS OF INTEREST

Fort Independence William J. Day Blvd., South Boston, MA 02127, 617-268-8870

Sullivan's Restaurant 2000 William J. Day Blvd.,
South Boston, MA 02127, 617-268-5685

ROUTE SUMMARY

1. Facing Fort Independence, take the path to the left (north side of the fort) to go around the fort clockwise.

2. One quarter of the way around the fort, go out on the pier on the left.

3. Retrace your steps back to the path and head south to cross the breakwater.

4. Once back on land, turn right to walk along Pleasure Bay back to your starting point.

Carson Beach

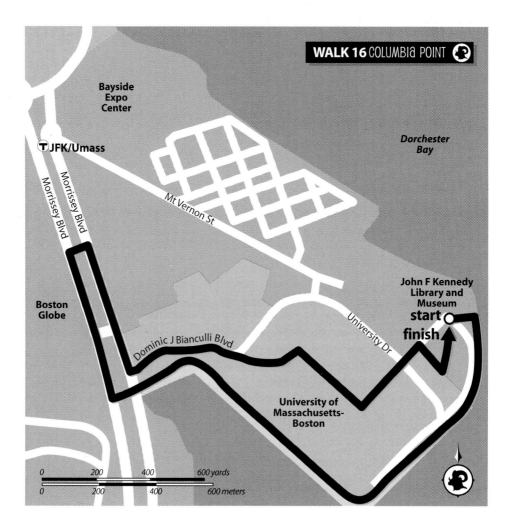

Bayside
Expo
Center

Dorchester
Bay

JFK/Umass

Mt Vernon St

Morrissey Blvd

Morrissey Blvd

Boston
Globe

John F Kennedy
Library and
Museum

start

finish

University Dr

Dominic J Bianculli Blvd

University of
Massachusetts-
Boston

0   200   400   600 yards
0   200   400   600 meters

16 COLUMBIA POINT: JFK LIBRARY AND UMASS BOSTON

BOUNDARIES: **Columbia Point Dr., University Dr. East, University Dr. South, William T. Morrissey Blvd.**
DISTANCE: **Approx. 2½ miles**
DIFFICULTY: **Easy**
PARKING: **There is free public parking at the John F. Kennedy Presidential Library and Museum.**
PUBLIC TRANSIT: **JFK/UMass T Station on the Red Line; busses 8 and 16**

Jutting into Dorchester Bay, the UMass Boston campus offers lovely views of Boston's south shore and the town of Quantum. But while the walk along the water is refreshing, even on the hottest of days, the real hero of this walk is the John F. Kennedy Presidential Library and Museum, a wonderful repository of not just presidential records but also an important collection of Ernest Hemingway's papers.

This is a great walk for late summer and fall, when the crisp air offers great views and the campus bustles with activity.

● Begin at the John F. Kennedy Presidential Library and Museum. Dedicated in 1979, the library's 21 permanent exhibits include archives, documents, and historic film reels that trace much of the life and career of America's 35th president. The library also houses the world's largest collection of Ernest Hemingway's papers and mementos. In addition, there is a cafe for a snack before you begin your walk. On any given day, you'll find a mix of serious scholars and groups of school kids and families on vacation.

After exploring the library, exit via the main doors. Take a moment to enjoy the stark white tower of the library. Designed by renowned architect I.M. Pei, the building is a dramatic shaft of white stucco and black glass.

● Facing the building, follow the patio down to the water, and then walk south on the Harborwalk. Here, you have splendid views of Dorchester Bay and Thompson Island, the long green island to the east, where Outward Bound holds programs, conferences, and team-building courses. To get closer to the water, you may want to walk out on the short pier with the yellow crane just south of the library.

- Follow the pathway around Columbia Point and walk south along the peninsula. The unnatural, geometric shape of Columbia Point is a sure tip-off to the fact that it was created from filled-in tidal flats.

- At the southern edge of the point, turn right to follow the peninsula back to the mainland.

- At the mainland, use the crosswalks to cross Morrissey Blvd. and turn right to head north on Morrissey. The large building on your left is the headquarters of the *Boston Globe*, long the dominant news rag of Beantown. The paper moved to this South Boston facility in 1958 after 87 years on Washington St. in downtown Boston. Free, hour-long tours of the plant and printing press are available, usually on Mondays and Thursdays, but it's best to call ahead for a reservation and specific times.

- Retrace your steps on Morrissey to Dominic J. Bianculli Blvd. and turn left to enter the UMass Boston campus. The school enrolls nearly 12,000 students in its many institutions, which include the Girl's High School for training teachers and an agricultural school. Established in 1964, it now boasts one of the most ethnically diverse student bodies in New England.

- Turn left on University Dr.

- Turn right on the path between the Healy Library and the Quinn Administration Building to head into the heart of the campus. Just past the Science Center is the Campus Center, opened in 2004. Stop in to check out the bulletin boards, use the bathroom, or grab a bite at the Atrium Cafe on the second floor.

- Exit the Campus Center through the same doors you entered and turn right to go north toward the JFK Library. You will pass a parking lot on the right and athletic fields with a track on the left.

- Directly across the parking lot from the JFK Library is the building of the Massachusetts Archives, at 220 Morrissey Blvd. Here, it's possible to research almost anything that has happened in Massachusetts in the last 400 years. With titles like *Volume 9: Domestic Relations, 1613* and *Volume 303: Petitions, 1659–1786*, the archives are exhaustive. The Commonwealth Museum, with exhibits on various aspects of life in the Commonwealth like the archaeology of the Big Dig and the role of democracy in Massachusetts, is in the same building.

● **Exit the Commonwealth Museum and cross the parking lot to return to the JFK Library.**

POINTS OF INTEREST

John F. Kennedy Presidential Library and Museum Columbia Point, Boston, MA 02125, 617-514-1600

***Boston Globe* headquarters** 135 Morrissey Blvd., Boston, MA 02125, 617-929-2000

UMass Boston 100 Morrissey Blvd., Boston, MA 02125, 617-287-5000

Massachusetts Archives 220 Morrissey Blvd., Boston, MA 02125, 617-727-2816

Commonwealth Museum 220 Morrissey Blvd., Boston, MA 02125, 617-727-9268

ROUTE SUMMARY

1. Begin at the JFK Library and walk to the water to follow the Harborwalk south around Columbia Point.

2. As you near the mainland, cross Morrissey Blvd. and turn right to follow Morrissey north.

3. Walk to the *Boston Globe* headquarters at 135 Morrissey Blvd.

4. Retrace your steps on Morrissey and turn left on Dominic J. Bianculli Blvd. to enter the UMass Boston campus.

5. Turn left on University Dr.

6. Turn right on the path between the Healy Library and the Quinn Administration Building.

7. From the Campus Center, go north to return to your starting point at the JFK Library.

JFK Library

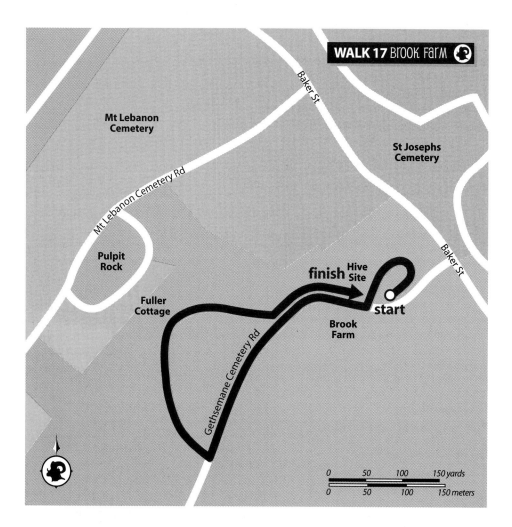

WALK 17 Brook Farm

Mt Lebanon
Cemetery

Baker St

St Josephs
Cemetery

Mt Lebanon Cemetery Rd

Pulpit
Rock

Baker St

finish   Hive
          Site

Fuller
Cottage

start

Brook
Farm

Gethsemane Cemetery Rd

0   50   100   150 yards
0   50   100   150 meters

17 Brook Farm: The Birds of Utopia

BOUNDARIES: **Baker St., Mt. Lebanon Cemetery, Mt. Lebanon Cemetery Rd., Gethsemane Cemetery Rd.**
DISTANCE: **Approx. 1 mile**
DIFFICULTY: **Moderate**
PARKING: **There is free parking at Brook Farm historical site.**
PUBLIC TRANSIT: **Bus 52**

In the first half of the 19th century, Boston was a hotbed of cultural activity, especially for transcendentalism, a loose set of beliefs and projects that emphasized humankind's inherent connection to God and to each other. This tour covers one of the most famous of the transcendentalist projects—an ill-fated utopian society known as Brook Farm. Beginning in 1841, a group of intellectuals and laborers followed the Unitarian minister and transcendentalist visionary George Ripley into the wilds of West Roxbury to live according to the ideals of transcendentalism and the practices set out by French utopian socialist Charles Fourier. Although the farm attracted the attention of Ralph Waldo Emerson and Henry David Thoreau and a young novelist named Nathaniel Hawthorne (who lived at the farm for half a year), it suffered an early demise in 1846 when its largest building burned to the ground. Now the 179-acre farm is protected as a National Historic Site and managed by the state Department of Conservation and Recreation.

This is a wonderful fall walk when the colors are on the trees and some of the underbrush has died away. Because paths can change from year to year and trail maintenance is sporadic at this site, actual conditions and directions may be slightly different from what is described here.

● Begin to the right of the parking area, at the Brook Farm National Historic Site display, where a kiosk offers some of the history and context of the farm. There's also a rough map here. The large barn to your left was not part of the original Brook Farm but was built on the site of the print shop for the *Harbinger*, a weekly journal edited by Brook Farm founder George Ripley. It dealt with mostly with social and educational issues, but also published poetry, music reviews, and news from Brook Farm.

- From the display, take the path leading to the right (northeast). As the path curves to the left, stop for a moment to gaze northwest across the field and down a short hill to the Mt. Lebanon Cemetery.

- Continue walking to head down this hill and across the street, where you will reach the site of the original school. Given its philosophical bent, it is not surprising that the community of Brook Farm was more successful with its education than its agriculture. There was a nursery school, primary school, and a college-preparatory program that sent many students to Harvard. Evening courses for the adults included classes on German, modern European history, and moral philosophy.

  Just out of view on your left is a huge rock formation accessible from the Mt. Lebanon Cemetery Rd. This rock was an integral part of the Brook Farm campus, and the group would often come here for Sunday church services. The rock also features in many scenes of Nathaniel Hawthorne's novel loosely based on his Brook Farm experience, *The Blithedale Romance*.

- Follow the path west toward the barn to the site of the Hive, a two-story farmhouse that served as the community's dining hall, library, and meeting room. After Brook Farm folded, the house was used periodically as an orphanage, but the house burned down in 1977. It is now just a peaceful spot in the woods.

- Return to the parking lot and turn right on the Gethsemane Cemetery access road.

- As you journey southwest on this road, look for the small plaque on the right-hand side. It honors the Second Massachusetts Infantry Regiment, which trained at the at the Brook Farm site (they called it "Camp Andrew") from 1861 to 1865, before shipping off to the Civil War.

- Continue on the access road another few hundred feet until a small parking area on the right and follow the trail leading out from the parking lot and into the woods. Just to the left of the path are the remains of the Margaret Fuller Cottage. Although

Back Story: Hawthorne the Farmer

In some ways, the writer Nathaniel Hawthorne's seven-month sojourn in West Roxbury reflects the trajectory of the entire experiment: early enthusiasm, weary contentment, growing disillusionment, and a disappointing exit.

He came to the farm cheerfully hoping to establish a peaceful home and enjoy an agrarian life among equals. In his first weeks, he worked with diligence and enthusiasm, milking cows, chopping hay, bringing in firewood, and pitching manure. A week later, he described himself as quite the farmer in his letters to his fiancée, Sophia: "It is an endless surprise to me how much work there is to be done in the world; but, thank God, I am able to do my share of it—and my ability increases daily. What a great, broad-shouldered, elephantine personage I shall become by and by."

But by midsummer, Hawthorne was singing a different tune. He complained that chopping wood disturbed "the equilibrium of the muscles and sinews," making it difficult for him to write. That minor complaint grew into full-blown hyperbole. "My soul obstinately refuses to be poured out on paper," he complained in his *American Notebooks*.

After a short break in September, he lasted until November when he had to sue Brook Farm to try to retrieve his initial investment.

Adapted from author Robert Todd Felton's book *A Journey into the Transcendentalists' New England* (Roaring Forties Press, 2006).

the transcendentalist writer and early feminist had no real intention of permanently joining the community, she was very supportive and visited often.

● Retrace your steps back to the parking lot, and turn left on the Gethsemane Cemetery access road to return to the start.

POINTS OF INTEREST

Brook Farm National Historic Site 670 Baker St., West Roxbury, MA 02132,
617-698-1802

route summary

1. Begin at the Brook Farm National Historic Site display and take the path leading to the right to make a counterclockwise loop (northeast) around the site of the original school, past the barn to the site of the Hive, a former two-story farmhouse that is now simply a peaceful spot in the woods.

2. Return to the parking lot and turn right to walk southeast on Gethsemane Cemetery Rd.

3. Turn right at the first parking lot on the right to follow the trail on a loop through the woods.

4. Retrace your steps to the parking lot and turn left (northwest) on Gethsemane Cemetery Rd. to return to your starting point.

Information kiosk, Brook Farm

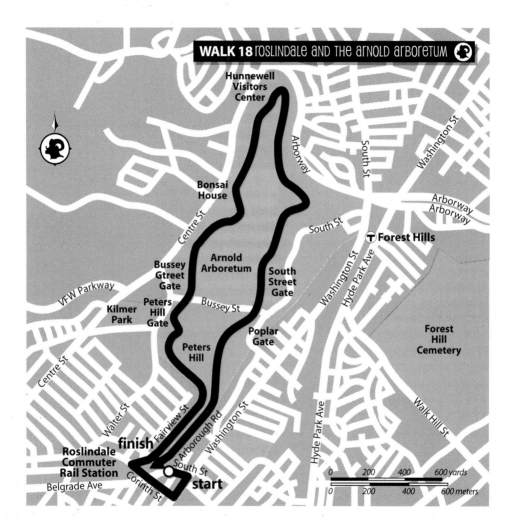

WALK 18 ROSLINDALE AND THE ARNOLD ARBORETUM

Hunnewell
Visitors
Center

Arborway

South St

Washington St

Arborway
Arborway

Bonsai
House

Centre St

South St

Ⓣ Forest Hills

Arnold
Arboretum

Bussey
Gtreet
Gate

South
Street
Gate

Washington St

Hyde Park Ave

VFW Parkway

Peters
Hill
Gate

Bussey St

Forest
Hill
Cemetery

Kilmer
Park

Poplar
Gate

Centre St

Peters
Hill

Walter St

Fairview St

S Arborough Rd

Washington St

Washington St

Hyde Park Ave

Walk Hill St

finish

0   200   400   600 yards

Roslindale
Commuter
Rail Station

South St

0   200   400   600 meters

Belgrade Ave

Corinth St

start

18 roslindale and the arnold arboretum: images of spring

BOUNDARIES: **Washington St., Corinth St., Centre St., Arborway**
DISTANCE: **Approx. 4½ miles**
DIFFICULTY: **Difficult**
PARKING: **Roslindale has a number of short-term parking lots on Tafthill Terrace and at the train station on Belgrade Ave. There are also a small number of parking spaces on the streets surrounding the arboretum.**
PUBLIC TRANSIT: **Roslindale train station on the commuter train Needham line; Forest Hills T Station on the Orange Line; busses 34, 35, 36, and 37**

Although this walk is mainly about the beautiful gardens of the Arnold Arboretum, it starts and ends in the charming nearby village of Roslindale, where you can grab a picnic lunch before the walk or an ice cream afterward.

The Arnold Arboretum's 256 acres of carefully managed plants (there are more than 15,000) are a welcome reprieve from the busy city any time of the year, but springtime trumps all other seasons. Choose your favorite flower, head to the arboretum when it is in bloom, and you won't be disappointed.

● **Begin at the Roslindale train station and head east on South St.**

● **Turn right on Poplar St. to enjoy Irving Adams Square (better known by the locals as Roslindale Square), named in honor of Massachusetts's first World War I casualty. The shops that line the square are a good indication of Roslindale's multi-ethnic population. Bakeries and dry cleaning services stand side by side with Thai restaurants and stores selling African goods. Roslindale, like many of the communities in this section of Boston, fell on tough times in the 1970s and '80s, but it has seen dramatic changes since the turn of the millennium. The city of Boston has made significant investments to revitalize Roslindale, spurring new businesses and attracting new residents.**

- Turn right on Corinth St. and walk west toward Fairview St. Pop into the Village Market at 30 Corinth to gather picnic food and swing by Solera, at 12 Corinth St., for the perfect bottle of wine to add to your basket.

  Go out the back door of Solera (or duck around the corner on Birch St.) to find Sophia's Grotto Cafe in a lovely brick courtyard with tables and flower plantings. Etched into granite panels along the alleyway connecting the courtyard with Birch St. are three excerpts of the Ithaca section of Homer's *Odyssey*. One is in Greek, one in Latin, and one is in English.

  If you are in more of a sandwich mood, try the Fornax Bread Company Incorporated, across the street from the Village Market, at 27 Corinth St.

- At the intersection of Corinth St. and Belgrade Ave., use the crosswalk to cross Belgrade to the sidewalk next to the train station parking lot.

- Turn left on the sidewalk and follow it around to the Alexander the Great Park. In the 1990s, the city of Athens, Greece, gave the city of Boston this park's 5-foot bronze statue of Alexander the Great. Continue along the sidewalk here to go under the railroad tracks (the road is Robert St., but there is no discernible street sign).

- Just after you go under the railroad tracks, take the first right you come to—a short-cut called S. Fairview St. This takes you north up the hill toward the arboretum. On the right, at the corner of S. Fairview and South St. (S. Fairview becomes Fairview St. here), is the Boston School of Modern Languages, housed in what was once the imposing Church of our Savior. Students come here from around the world to brush up on their English.

- Continue on Fairview St. until it dead-ends at the arboretum (Mendum St. branches off to the left).

- Head through the Mendum St. gate and turn left on Peters Hill Rd. to explore the Arnold Arboretum, the oldest public arboretum in North America. Founded by whaling merchant James Arnold, the Arnold Arboretum of Harvard University was given to Harvard in 1872. The 256-acre park was designed by Frederick Law Olmsted and

Charles Sprague Sargent, the arboretum's first director. In 1882, the land was given back to the city of Boston, which granted Harvard a thousand-year lease.

- Near the crest of the hill, turn right on a footpath leading to a sweeping vista of the city. You can easily make out the Prudential Center and Hancock Tower of distant Boston. Return via the path to Peters Hill Rd. to continue heading north. As you begin to head down the other side of the hill, look to the left for the tulip trees just past the old burying ground.

- Turn left at the first junction you encounter. This paved road leads to the Peters Hill gate. Just past the gate is busy Bussey St.

- Cross Bussey St. at the crosswalk, turn left on Hemlock Hill Rd., and look for Conifer Path immediately on the right.

- Turn right (north) on Conifer Path, which winds through a forest of bamboo (on the left) and fir (on the right), before bearing north again near a grove of hickories and silverbells. The path dumps you onto Valley Rd.

- Turn left (north) on Valley Rd. and continue to where it merges with Bussey Hill Rd. near the Centre St. gate.

- Continue north on Bussey Hill Rd. and look for signs on your left leading to the Dana Greenhouses. Take the path up, and stop at the Bonsai House to view the Larz Anderson Bonsai Collection, which is one of the oldest bonsai collections in America and boasts more than 30 bonsai trees from around the world. Larz Anderson was the American

Magnolia trees in full bloom at Arnold Arboretum Hunnewell Visitors Center ambassador to Japan and brought many of these "dwarf trees" back from Japan in 1913. In the winter, they are put into cold storage for protection.

- From the bonsai collection, follow the Bridal Path north to the Hunnewell Visitors Center, a lovely facility with exhibits, a gift shop, and restrooms. The center also offers courses in everything from planting Chinese tree peonies to garden and landscape writing.

- From the visitors center, head south on Meadow Rd., which leads past a garden of magnolias and tulips and then swings south toward the Bradley Collection of Rosaceous Plants (that which we call a rose, which, of course, by any other name would smell as sweet . . .). If you are concerned, ask the friendly staff at the visitors center for directions before you leave.

- Just south of the rose garden, where Meadow Rd. meets Forest Hills and Bussey Hill roads, bear right on Bussey Hill Rd.

- Take an immediate left on the Beech Path, which leads down to the Asian collection, with its remarkable, white-leaved dove tree, a Korean stewartia, and a paperbark maple.

- Walk past the Asian collection to a stand of silver-barked birches, and then turn left on Valley Rd. to head down past the rhododendrons to the South St. gate.

- Turn right on South St., which brings you past Bussey St. and the Poplar St. gate to Peters Hill Rd.

- About halfway up the hill, bear left on the path that leads to the smaller gate just down the hill from the Mendum Gate you entered. Exit through this gate and walk south on Arborough Rd.

POINTS OF INTEREST

Village Market 30 Corinth St., Roslindale, MA 02131, 617-327-2588

Solera 12 Corinth St., Roslindale, MA 02131, 617-469-4005

Sophia's Grotto Cafe 22 Birch St., Roslindale, MA 02131, 617-323-4595

Fornax Bread Company Incorporated 27 Corinth St., Roslindale, MA 02131, 617-325-8852

Boston School of Modern Languages 814 South St., Roslindale, MA 02131, 617-325-2760

Arnold Arboretum Hunnewell Visitors Center 125 Arborway, Jamaica Plain, MA 02130, 617-524-1718.

route summary

1. Begin at the Roslindale train station and walk east on South St.
2. Turn right on Poplar St.
3. Turn right on Corinth St.
4. Cross Belgrade Ave. at the crosswalk and turn left to follow sidewalk under train tracks.
5. Turn right on S. Fairview St.
6. Enter the Arnold Arboretum through the Mendum St. gate.
7. Turn left on Peters Hill Rd.
8. At junction with other leg of Peters Hill Rd., turn left.
9. Cross Bussey St. at the crosswalk, follow the walkway to Hemlock Hill Rd., and turn left.
10. Turn right on Conifer Path.
11. Turn left on Valley Rd., and then merge with Bussey Hill Rd. near the Centre St. gate.
12. Turn left on the path leading to Bonsai House.
13. Just past Bonsai House, follow the Bridal Path to the Hunnewell Visitors Center.
14. From the visitors center, follow Meadow Rd. south.
15. Bear right on Bussey Hill Rd.
16. Turn left on Beech Path.
17. Turn left on Valley Rd.
18. Turn right on South St.
19. Turn left on Peters Hill Rd.
20. Exit the arboretum at the gate below the Mendum St. Gate.
21. Walk south on Arborough Rd.
22. Turn left on South St. to return to the Roslindale train station.

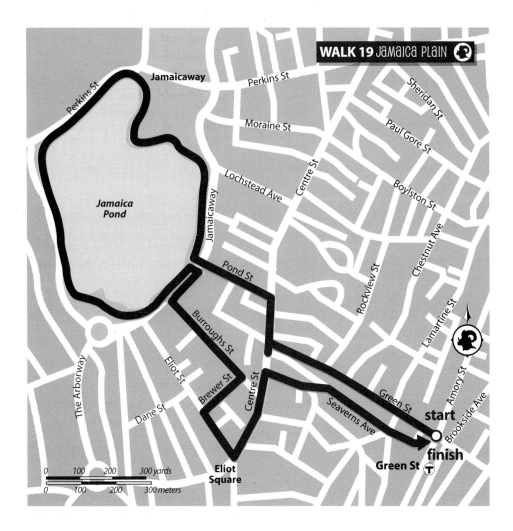

Perkins St

Jamaicaway

Perkins St

Moraine St

Sheridan St

Paul Gore St

Lochstead Ave

Centre St

Boylston St

Jamaica
Pond

Jamaicaway

Chestnut Ave

Pond St

Rockview St

Lamartine St

Burroughs St

The Arborway

Eliot St

Brewer St

Centre St

Green St

Amory St

Dane St

Seaverns Ave

Brookside Ave

start

Eliot
Square

finish

Green St Ⓣ

0   100   200   300 yards

0   100   200   300 meters

19 Jamaica Plain: Zaim's Most Famous Walking Tour*

BOUNDARIES: **Perkins St., Centre St., Arborway, Francis Parkman Dr., Amory St.**
DISTANCE: **Approx. 3 miles (with possible nearly 2-mile extension around Leverett Pond)**
DIFFICULTY: **Easy**
PARKING: **There is a large, free, two-hour lot on Burroughs St. and limited free parking on Eliot St., Centre St., and South St.**
PUBLIC TRANSIT: **Green St. T Station on the Orange Line; busses 38, 39, 41, 42, and 48**

Zaim is a 7-year-old friend of mine who happens to be a Jamaica Plain expert. He helped me design this tour of J.P. (as it's called throughout Boston), including the best spots for watching trains, skipping rocks at Jamaica Pond, and, of course, eating ice cream. His mother helped fill in the rest. J.P. got its start as a farming community and then a comfortable Victorian suburb of Boston. Jamaica Plain fell on harder times in the 1970s and '80s, when the real estate prices tanked and many of the stores boarded up. But fueled by a revived economy and soaring real estate prices downtown, J.P. is now a hip and multicultural neighborhood, boasting internet cafes and eclectic stores along Centre St.

With flowers blooming along the pond and children getting ready for summer, spring is a great season for this walk.

- **Begin at the Green St. T Station at the corner of Woolsey Square and Green St. On the opposite side of Green is a wide open platform Zaim loves for viewing the commuter trains and the Orange Line subway trains rumbling through. If you're lucky, the Acela train from New York City will speed by, too. Walk west on Green St.**

- **To get you started on the right foot, turn left on Centre St. and go half a block to J.P. Licks. The Boston-area ice cream institution is in the renovated 1800s-era firehouse and has a wonderful patio for enjoying your ice cream. Check out the**

---

* Special thanks to Zaim Elkalai and his mother, Kathleen Traphagen.

chalkboard for the best in impromptu children's art. When you are ready to move on, turn left out of J.P. Licks to head north on Centre St.

- Turn left on Pond St. and follow it to Jamaica Pond. After you cross the Jamaicaway (carefully), continue straight to the boathouse, where you can rent a boat from the Courageous Sailing Center, get something to eat at the snack bar (note that the hours are sometimes erratic), or check out the Jamaica Pond Nature Center, run by the Boston Park Rangers. The displays will help you find the turtles, frogs, herons, and barred owls that make their home in and around the 68-acre "kettle" pond—one of the many ponds in Massachusetts that formed in a natural depression left when the ice age glaciers receded. There is fishing in the pond but no swimming.

- Take a right on the path to walk around the pond counterclockwise. At the northeast corner of the lake (just before the lakeside trail curves to the left), the trail splits at a Y junction. If you turn right here, the trail will take you down the Jamaicaway, crossing Perkins St. and Willow Pond Rd., before circling Leverett Pond and returning. This extension would add up to about 2 miles, depending on which trails you use. Jamaica Pond and the Jamaicaway down to Leverett Pond are integral links in the 1,100-acre chain of parks that comprise landscape architect Frederick Law Olmsted's "Emerald Necklace," which is popular with runners and joggers.

- To continue on this walk, take a left at the Y junction and continue around the pond until Burroughs St. As the path parallels Perkins St. on the western side of the pond, the trail runs close to the water. This is one of Zaim's favorite places to come skip stones. See if you can beat seven.

- As the path returns to the starting point, cross Jamaicaway at the crosswalk near Pond St. and turn right to go back one block to Burroughs St.

- Turn left on Burroughs St., which provides an excellent example of the well-preserved Victorian houses that make up the gentry of Jamaica Plain.

- Turn right on Brewer St. The Brewer St. Tot Lot, on the left side, about halfway down Brewer St., received a favorable review from Zaim for being a nice, quiet playground—although he is now a little too grown up for it. He told me it is better for the younger kids.

● Continue down Brewer and turn left on Eliot St., one of the nicest streets in Jamaica Plain, and maybe all of Boston. Quiet and well-shaded, it is also full of history. For example, at 24 Eliot, at the intersection of Brewer and Eliot, is the cheery, bright yellow Eliot School schoolhouse. The school was founded in 1676 to educate both the Puritans and Native Americans. It's now the Eliot School of Fine and Applied Arts, which offers courses in things like painting, sewing, and drawing. It is particularly well known for the master classes in woodworking and furniture design. For example, Zaim's dad made an art table for him in a woodworking class here.

Along Eliot, you also have the chance to enjoy a few of the lovely Gothic, Victorian, and Italianate designs of buildings. On the left side, at 15–21 Eliot, is a row of lovely Victorian shingle houses painted in vibrant purples and browns, with white trim. Just past those houses is the Greek Revival-style Eliot Hall (7A Eliot), home to the Footlight Club. The Footlight Club was founded in 1877, making it the oldest amateur theatrical club in the United States. The club moved into this hall in 1878 and is still entertaining audiences with quality plays like *All My Sons* and *West Side Story*. Almost directly across the street from the Eliot Hall is the First Church in Jamaica Plain, built in 1853. Its grey solidity anchors the south end of J.P.'s commercial district.

● Turn left on Centre St. and follow it to Seaverns Ave. This section of Centre is rife with wonderful places. Zaim suggests Boing!, at 729 Centre, for toys. Boing! was started in October of 2000 and is the type of toy store you wish you had in your town. Poke your head in to check out the wide variety of educational toys and handcrafted goodies, in addition to a few of the old standbys like Legos. If you need some food at this point, try Wonder Spice Cafe, at 697 Centre St. It serves mostly Cambodian dishes, as well as some Thai and "create your own dish" options.

● Turn right on Seaverns Ave. and follow it to the Green St. T Station.

POINTS OF INTEREST

J.P. Licks 659 Centre St., Jamaica Plain, MA 02130, 617-524-6740

Courageous Sailing Center Jamaica Pond Boathouse, Jamaica Plain, MA 02130, 617-522-5061

Jamaica Pond Nature Center Jamaica Pond Boathouse, Jamaica Plain, MA 02130, 617-522-5061

Brewer St. Tot Lot Brewer St. between Burroughs St. and Thomas St., Jamaica Plain, MA 02130

Eliot School of Fine and Applied Arts 24 Eliot St., Jamaica Plain, MA 02130, 617-524-3313

Footlight Club 7A Eliot St., Jamaica Plain, MA 02130, 617-524-6506

Boing! 729 Centre St., Jamaica Plain, MA 02130, 617-522-7800

Wonder Spice Cafe 697 Centre St., Jamaica Plain, MA 02130, 617-522-020

ROUTE SUMMARY

1. Begin at the Green St. T Station at the corner of Woolsey Square and Green St. and walk west on Green.
2. Turn right on Centre St.
3. Turn left on Pond St.
4. Turn right to go around the pond counterclockwise.
5. As the path returns to the starting point, cross Jamaicaway at the crosswalk near Pond St. and turn right to go back one block on Jamaicaway to Burroughs St.
6. Turn left on Burroughs St.
7. Turn right on Brewer St.
8. Turn left on Eliot St.
9. Turn left on Centre St.
10. Turn right on Seaverns Ave. and follow it to the Green St. T Station

Mural at the corner of Hall and Centre streets

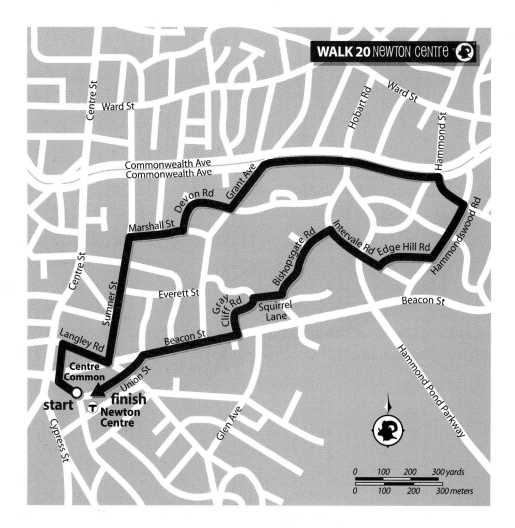

Centre St

Ward St

Commonwealth Ave
Commonwealth Ave

Hobart Rd

Ward St

Hammond St

Devon Rd

Grant Ave

Marshall St

Centre St

Sumner St

Everett St

Bishopsgate Rd

Intervale Rd

Edge Hill Rd

Hammondswood Rd

Gray Cliff Rd

Squirrel Lane

Beacon St

Langley Rd

Beacon St

Centre Common

Union St

start

finish
Newton Centre

Cypress St

Glen Ave

Hammond Pond Parkway

0   100   200   300 yards

0   100   200   300 meters

20 NEWTON CENTRE: HEARTBREAK HILL AND HAMMOND'S ORCHARDS

BOUNDARIES: Commonwealth Ave., Hammondswood Rd., Beacon St., Centre St.
DISTANCE: Approx. 2½ miles
DIFFICULTY: Moderate
PARKING: There is free, two-hour parking in the lot on Langley Rd., at the intersection of Beacon St. and Langley, and metered spaces are along Beacon St., Centre St., and Commonwealth Ave.
PUBLIC TRANSIT: Newton Centre T Station on the Green Line; bus 52

Newton Centre is a classic well-heeled Boston suburb—quiet and sleepy but with an eclectic mix of shops and restaurants. It has a carefully preserved quaintness that still buzzes with day-to-day activity. The surrounding neighborhoods mix traditional Victorian shingle houses with neatly maintained ranch houses, all on quiet side streets that are great for walking.

Add in some fall foliage and the humming sounds of leaf blowers, and this is the perfect way to spend a fall day in New England.

● This is one walk where the starting point is a destination in itself. The Newton Centre T Station is a delightful little station built according to Boston architect H.H. Richardson's Romanesque designs (he died before it could be completed) in 1886. Stop to admire the rough-hewn stone construction with the alternating colors before setting out on your journey.

From the Newton Centre T Station, head west on Union St. to go clockwise around the Union Building, which was built in 1896 as a commercial space and meeting hall. It now houses a number of trendy clothing boutiques. The next building over, Bray's Block or Bray's Hall, was constructed just three years before (in 1893 also as a mixed-use building), but this one also had a bowling alley and indoor tennis court. It's a good example of Classical Revival style, and has been noted for the dormers, masonry work, and copper-clad roof.

- Follow Union St. as it curves around the west end of the Union Building, and becomes Herrick Rd. Follow the sidewalk out to Beacon St. and use the crosswalk to cross Beacon.

- Once across Beacon, enter the Centre Common flower garden (above the parking lot) to enjoy the profusion of color. The trees were planted here in 1880 by the Newton Centre Improvement Association, and the garden blooms almost year-round. Across Centre St. are ornamentations of a different sort—a number of high-end clothing stores and little boutiques line the northern side of Centre St.

- From the northwest corner of the garden, turn right at the tiled art sculpture on the corner of Langley Rd. and cross to the northern side of the street, where all the shops are. If you're hungry, try Johnny's Luncheonette (30 Langley Rd.), Newton Centre's version of a greasy spoon. If you suddenly need a rainbow-colored afro or some fake blood, or maybe silly party tricks, stop into the Party Shop (42 Langley Rd.), just one door down. It's a pretty fun place.

- At the end of the block, where Langley, Sumner St., and Beacon St. converge, make a sharp left on Sumner and head north. Once the railways were introduced to Boston, Newton grew from a farming outpost into a commuter suburb, and Sumner was one of the first streets to be developed—the lots were snapped up by the wealthiest families first. As a result, the houses here are both historic and large. Well-maintained examples of Victorian and Colonial Revival homes line both sides of the street, with most dating back to the late 19th century. On the right, at 180 Sumner, is a great example of shingle-style architecture. For stick-style houses with decorative wood finishes, see the houses at 166 and 147 Sumner.

- After three blocks, turn right on Marshall St. to walk through the heart of Newton Centre's residential neighborhood. If you are here on a weekday, the place will be silent except perhaps for the buzzing of leaf blowers. There are also a set of burning bushes (for those from outside the area, these are not the Bible's burning bushes, but a real plant that turns fiery red in the fall) along here that are truly spectacular come October.

- Turn left on Devon Rd.

Back Story: Boston Marathon

In 1896, members of the Boston Athletic Association attended the first modern Olympic Games, held in Athens, Greece. They did well in many of the events, except for one they hadn't seen before: a long-distance footrace called a "marathon." They brought the idea back to Boston and ran the first one in April of 1897 (the first in the country had been run the year before from Connecticut to New York City), with 15 men who ran 24.5 miles from the Boston suburb of Ashland to Exeter St. in Back Bay.

Since then, the Boston Marathon has become one of the country's most prestigious marathons. It is the oldest marathon run continuously, the oldest run on the same course each year (with a few slight modifications), and one of the only marathons in the world for which you have to qualify.

Women were not officially accepted until 1972, but in 1966, that didn't stop Roberta Gibb, who hid in the bushes until the start and then ran without a number. The very next year, Kathrine Switzer obtained an official race number and ran under the gender-neutral name "K. Switzer." Race officials tried to physically remove her from the course, but she persevered and finished the race.

Another famous woman runner, though, did not actually run the whole thing. Rosie Ruiz jumped onto the course with a mile left and sprinted to the end to take the 1980 women's title. However, people started to question this amateur runner who had bested the competition so soundly, apparently without even breaking a sweat. Her title was stripped eight days later.

● **Turn left on Grant Ave.**

● **Turn right on Commonwealth Ave. If you listen carefully along here, you might hear the sound of sneakers on pavement and labored breathing. This section of Commonwealth is known as "Heartbreak Hill" to those who follow the Boston Marathon. The hill is a slight, half-mile rise, but, for the runners who have come 20.5 miles to get to this point, it's a heartbreaker. From the top of the hill, runners are** greeted with the Boston College marching band, lots of cheering, and the message, "It's all downhill from here!" So, unless you've been training, avoid this walk on the third Monday of April, when the Boston Marathon is part of the Patriot's Day celebration.

● You are not going downhill yet. Turn right on Hammond St. (just past Wachusett Rd.) and wander down to Hammondswood Rd. If you're noticing a trend—yes, the Hammond family was prominent in Newton Centre's history. Little could Thomas Hammond have imagined what a real-estate feat he had achieved in the mid-1630s. He and a partner had purchased several hundred acres of fertile land, in what is now this highly sought after suburb of Boston. For several generations, the Hammond family lived, farmed, and made their mark in Newton, lending the family name to a pond, woods, and numerous streets in the area.

● Turn right on Hammondswood.

● Turn right on Edge Hill Rd.

● Turn right on Intervale Rd.

● Turn left on Bishopsgate Rd. and follow it until you encounter what may look like a driveway, but is in fact Squirrel Ln.

● Turn right on Squirrel Ln, a small unpaved road that is not much more than a gravel path. The sign here—NOT A PUBLIC WAY, DANGEROUS—is meant for cars; on foot, you are more than safe.

● Turn left on Gray Cliff Rd. and follow the sounds of cars down the hill.

● Turn right on Beacon St. and cross the street at the crosswalk where Dalton Rd. comes in from the right.

● Bear left on Union St. to return to the Newton Centre T Station. If you'd like to finish off with a cappuccino and a cookie, continue west on Beacon to the Peet's Coffee and Tea on the left, where locals curl up on chairs near the windows. Or bear right on Langley Rd. to do a little shopping before turning left on Union St.

POINTS OF INTEREST

Johnny's Luncheonette 30 Langley Rd., Newton, MA 02459, 617-527-3223
Party Shop Incorporated 42 Langley Rd., Newton, MA 02459, 617-244-8382
Peet's Coffee and Tea 776 Beacon St., Newton, MA 02459, 617-244-1577

ROUTE SUMMARY

1.   From the Newton Centre T Station, walk west on Union St., which becomes Herrick Rd.
2.   Cross Beacon St. and follow the sidewalk on the left side of the parking lot toward the flower gardens above the parking lot.
3.   Turn right into the gardens to follow the path running parallel to Centre St.
3.   Turn right on Langley Rd.
4.   At the intersection of Langley, Beacon St., and Sumner St., make a sharp left on Sumner.
5.   Turn right on Marshall St.
6.   Turn left on Devon Rd.
7.   Turn left on Grant Ave.
8.   Turn right on Commonwealth Ave.
9.   Turn right on Hammond St.
10. Turn right on Hammondswood Rd.
11. Turn right on Edge Hill Rd.
12. Turn right on Intervale Rd.
13. Turn left on Bishopsgate Rd.
14. Turn right on Squirrel Ln.
15. Turn left on Gray Cliff Rd.
16. Turn right on Beacon St.
17. Turn left on Union St. to return to the Newton Centre T Station.

The Victorian houses of Sumner St.

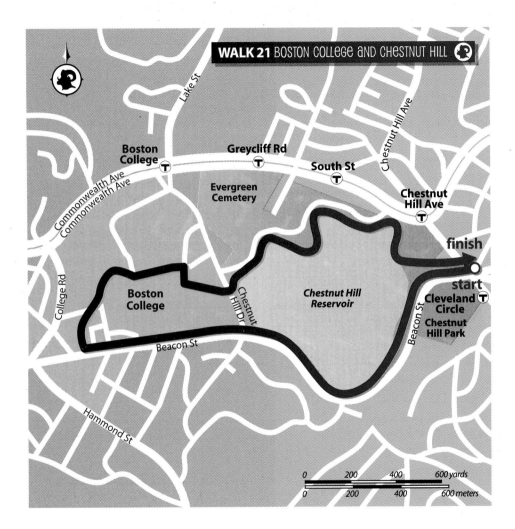

WALK 21 BOSTON COLLEGE AND CHESTNUT HILL

Lake St

Boston
College Ⓣ

Greycliff Rd Ⓣ

Chestnut Hill Ave

South St Ⓣ

Commonwealth Ave
Commonwealth Ave

Evergreen
Cemetery

Chestnut
Hill Ave Ⓣ

finish

College Rd

Boston
College

Chestnut
Hill Dr

Chestnut Hill
Reservoir

Beacon St

start

Cleveland
Circle Ⓣ

Chestnut
Hill Park

Beacon St

Hammond St

| 0 | 200 | 400 | 600 yards |
| 0 | 200 | 400 | 600 meters |

21 BOSTON COLLEGE AND CHESTNUT HILL: OF EAGLES AND CHESTNUTS

BOUNDARIES: **Commonwealth Ave., Beacon St., College Rd., Chestnut Hill Dr.**
DISTANCE: **Approx. 3 miles**
DIFFICULTY: **Moderate**
PARKING: **There is free two-hour parking along Commonwealth Ave. and free three-hour parking along Beacon St., by the reservoir.**
PUBLIC TRANSIT: **Cleveland Circle T Station on the Green Line (C branch); busses 51 and 86**

Boston is nothing if not a college town. With nearly 40 colleges and universities, academic campuses are easy to come by. But Boston College is unique for its wooded hills, pleasant reservoir, and glimpse of the Boston skyline. Founded in 1863 by the Society of Jesus, Boston College opened in 1864 with a mere three teachers and 22 students. By the beginning of the 20th century, the school had outgrown its Boston campus and construction of the Chestnut Hill campus began in 1909. By 1913, the college had opened the first building on the new campus, Gasson Hall, and moved completely out of Boston. Today, the Chestnut Hill campus covers 117 acres, and Boston College has 675 faculty and more than 14,000 students.

Combine this walk with a football game in the fall, when the air is crisp and student fans in their maroon and gold give the whole area an electric charge. Although this tour winds through the center of campus, you may want to spend more time exploring the corners of the campus as well. Stop by the Admissions Office in Devlin Hall for more information and guided tours.

● From the Cleveland Circle T Station, navigate the maze of crosswalks to the northern side of Beacon St. and head west.

● Just past the community center on the right, bear right on the path that leads up to the water, and once at the water, turn left to go along the southern shore of the reservoir.

The area here is known as the Chestnut Hill Reservation, a parcel of land and water listed on the National Register of Historic Places and is also a City of Boston Landmark. Formerly a swampy marsh and meadowland, the land was transformed in 1867 when the local water authority built a 37.5-acre reservoir called Lawrence Basin. A second, much larger reservoir, the 87.5-acre Bradlee Basin, was built a few years later in 1870. Together, these two basins (known as the Chestnut Hill Reservoir) distributed water to downtown Boston until the mid-20th century, when the Lawrence Basin was phased out and filled in. Boston College's stadium is now on that site. Bradlee Basin was taken off-line in 1970 and has become the centerpiece of the Chestnut Hill Reservation and renamed the Chestnut Hill Reservoir.

Although created for a utilitarian purpose, the Chestnut Hill Reservation has a long legacy as a recreational destination. When the basins were constructed, an 80-foot-wide path was also put in and it quickly became a popular place for "pleasure drives" (part of that road is still being used as Chestnut Hill Dr. today). A decorative iron fence was added in 1928 to prevent people from dumping their garbage in the water. The reservoir continues to be a popular place for serious runners, casual dog walkers, and friends out picnicking. About halfway around the southern side (where the shoreline swings northwest for a bit), turn around to catch a glimpse of the Prudential Tower and the John Hancock Tower.

● Continue along the southern side to the western edge of the reservoir, and leave the waterside to cross Chestnut Hill Dr. and continue up the hill on Beacon St.

● Just past Campion Hall on the right, turn right on the campus road to enter the Boston College campus. Directly ahead of you is a roundabout and a quad to the right of Fulton Hall. Enter this quad (the grass is in more of an oval shape than the traditional rectangle) and take the path on the eastern side of Fulton Hall.

● Turn left just past Fulton Hall to enter the main quad. Standing in the middle of the quad, facing north, you will see Gasson Hall directly ahead, Lyons Hall to the left, Devlin Hall to the right, and Fulton Hall behind you. On any given day during the school year, this quad could be packed with students advocating for some cause, admiring an art exhibition, or just hanging out.

- From the main quad, walk north to Gasson Hall, the oldest building (and B.C.'s signature hall) on campus. Venture inside for a peak at the classical paintings and sculptures that decorate the central rotunda; the inspirational sayings on these pieces of art provide a nice contrast to the cold Gothic stonework.

- From Gasson Hall, cross the large cement plaza and head east to the O'Neill Library. This plaza, with its broad cement risers, was designed as a central meeting place and open-air auditorium. It has hosted public ceremonies, concerts, theater presentations, and even pep rallies. The plaza is named after former Speaker of the House and Boston College alum, Thomas "Tip" O'Neill. In a campus full of Gothic arches and granite towers, the modern lines and concrete construction of the library stick out like a sore thumb.

- Skip looking inside the drab and uninspiring library, and head down the wide staircase that bisects the building and takes you underneath the library.

- The stairs end at a walkway behind the library; turn right here and walk 200 feet for a great view of B.C.'s Conte Forum and Alumni Stadium. Alumni Stadium opened in 1957 with a game against the U.S. Navy, and since then has hosted thousands of screaming Eagles fans cheering their surprisingly successful football team with floods of maroon and gold.

- Continue along the path and take the first staircase on the left down to the Edmond Roadway (also called Campanella Way), which leads past the stadium and the baseball fields until it reaches Chestnut Hill Dr.

- Cross Chestnut Hill Dr. (carefully, cars can go fast through here) and turn left at the water to resume your trip around the northern edge of the reservoir. This quiet section offers peaceful views across the lake.

- From the gatehouse, turn left to follow Beacon St. back to the Cleveland Circle T Station.

POINTS OF INTEREST

Chestnut Hill Reservation Chestnut Hill Dr. and Beacon St., Allston/Brighton, MA 02134, 617-333-7404

Boston College 140 Commonwealth Ave., Chestnut Hill, MA 02467, 617-552-3100

route summary

1. From the Cleveland Circle T Station, cross to the northern side of Beacon St. and walk west on Beacon.

2. Just past the community center, bear right on the path that leads up to the reservoir, and then turn left to walk clockwise around the lake.

3. At the western edge of the lake, leave the waterside to cross Chestnut Hill Dr. and continue up the hill on Beacon St.

4. At Campion Hall, turn right to enter the Boston College campus.

5. Enter the quad to the right of Fulton Hall and take the path on the eastern side of Fulton.

6. Just past Fulton Hall, turn left to enter the main quad and walk north to Gasson Hall.

7. From Gasson Hall, cross the plaza east to the O'Neill Library.

8. From the O'Neill Library, descend the stairs that go under the building.

9. Turn right on the path behind the library and then make a quick left to go down the stairs to the Conte Forum and Alumni Stadium.

10. At the bottom of the stairs, follow Edmond Roadway (also called Campanella Way) to Chestnut Hill Dr.

11. Cross Chestnut Hill Dr. and turn left to walk clockwise around the reservoir to the gatehouse.

12. From the gatehouse, turn left to follow Beacon St. back to the Cleveland Circle T Station.

Boston College

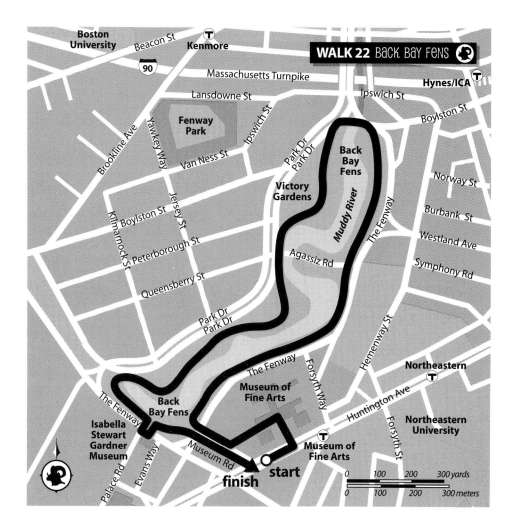

Boston University

Beacon St

Kenmore

90

Massachusetts Turnpike

Ipswich St

Hynes/ICA

Lansdowne St

Boylston St

Fenway Park

Ipswich St

Park Dr
Park Dr

Back Bay Fens

Norway St

Brookline Ave

Yawkey Way

Van Ness St

Victory Gardens

Muddy River

The Fenway

Burbank St

Westland Ave

Boylston St

Jersey St

Agassiz Rd

Symphony Rd

Kilmarnock St

Peterborough St

Queensberry St

Park Dr
Park Dr

The Fenway

Forsyth Way

Hemenway St

Northeastern

The Fenway

Back Bay Fens

Museum of Fine Arts

Huntington Ave

Forsyth St

Northeastern University

Isabella Stewart Gardner Museum

Evans Way

Museum Rd

Museum of Fine Arts

finish   start

Palace Rd

0   100   200   300 yards
0   100   200   300 meters

22 Back Bay Fens: Fine Art Along the Muddy River

BOUNDARIES: Fenway, Park Dr., Huntington Ave.
DISTANCE: Approx. 2¼ miles
DIFFICULTY: Easy
PARKING: There is limited paid parking in the garage on Museum Rd. and in the adjacent lot.
PUBLIC TRANSIT: MFA T Station on the Green Line (E branch); bus 39

Combining three great art collections with cheerful park strolls and a bit of history, this walk begins at the Museum of Fine Arts and wanders the paths of the Back Bay Fens, a bucolic park lining the banks of the Muddy River. The route returns via Huntington Ave. and the Massachusetts College of Art, with a stop for afternoon tea at the Isabella Stewart Gardner Museum.

Springtime brings the Kelleher Rose Garden and the Fenway Victory Gardens to life. Afternoons and evenings offer long light and the crack of a bat with cheering crowds to accompany your perambulations.

● Begin at the MFA T Station on Huntington Ave., cross Huntington to stand in front of the huge Museum of Fine Arts, which houses more than 450,000 objects. Its grey arms stretch out to invite you into the central courtyard. And if that doesn't draw you in, the outspread arms of the Cyrus Dallin statue in the front courtyard, *Appeal to the Great Spirit*, definitely will. Housing John Singer Sargent portraits, Paul Revere's silverwork, and an outstanding Asian collection, this museum is far too much to do in one day. Pick one collection or join one of the guided tours, which start at 10:30 AM and run throughout each day.

● Leave the museum through the bookstore door and turn right on Museum Rd. to reach the Back Bay Fens. Be careful crossing Fenway to reach the park paths—there's not a crosswalk here.

● Turn right on the path to go around the Fens counterclockwise. In 1879, Frederick Law Olmsted designed a series of connected parks in Boston called the "Emerald Necklace." One of the finest is the Back Bay Fens, a winding park through what once was a tidal marsh, and later was a polluted wetland. The park has evolved considerably since Olmsted's original creation. Both formal and community gardens have been added, ball fields created, and memorials built. Although slow-moving Muddy River, which flows down the center of the park, tends to get a little murky come late summer, the cool shade provides relief on hot days.

● At the north end of the Fens, follow the path up on to Boylston St. and bear left on Boylston to cross a bridge. From the bridge, you can look up the Muddy River to the south.

● After the bridge, turn left on the first path you come to and walk straight to the Fenway Victory Gardens, the last remaining World War II community garden in the country (nearly 22 million Americans planted a victory garden during World War II). Competition is fierce for these small garden plots, and residents often seek to outdo each other with their horticultural acumen. Choose any of the paths that lead through the

Back Story:
Frederick Law Olmsted

Beginning in 1875, famed landscape architect Frederick Law Olmsted had a hand in the creation of most outdoor spaces in Boston. Designer of Boston's "Emerald Necklace" series of interconnected parks linking Jamaica Plain with the Charles River Esplanade, Olmsted and his firm (which included his sons) helped design the Arnold Arboretum, Franklin Park, the Charles River Esplanade, the Public Garden, and the North End playground.

In addition to his work in Boston, Olmsted worked hard to protect Niagara Falls, preserve Yosemite National Park, design New York City's Central Park, and create Washington D.C.'s Capitol grounds. In total, his firm was involved with nearly 5,000 projects in 45 states. Olmsted liked to create natural settings that were as practical and accessible as they were beautiful.

Back Story: The Case Of The Empty Art Displays

One of the stipulations in Isabella Stewart Gardner's will was that all the art in the Isabella Stewart Gardner Museum be left exactly where she hung it—not a piece should be moved. Unfortunately, thieves did not heed her desires, and in 1990, they stole paintings by Vermeer, Rembrandt, Degas, and Manet, as well other works and artifacts totaling nearly $300 million. Although the FBI continues to work on the case (and has offered a reward of $5 million just in case you've got a hot tip), the art has never been returned. And, to top it all off, because of Gardner's stipulation that the museum remain exactly as she left it, the spaces where the stolen art used to hang remain empty to this day.

7 acres of individual plots or admire them from the outside by taking the path that bears to the left near the water.

● After the gardens, bend around the water on the path that goes near Park Dr. and then veers to the left again. On your left are the World War II, Vietnam, and Korean War memorials, as well as the Kelleher Rose Garden, a stunning bed with roses of every shape, color, and size lining the circular paths. (If you like the smell of roses, visit in June, when hundreds of roses bloom.)

● From the rose garden, take the path leading due west, toward the tennis courts, and then bear left to follow the path between the track and the Muddy River.

● As the path curves around to the right and heads north again, you come to a paved street (Fenway) that cuts across the Fens. Bear left here to loop around and start back down the Muddy River along the southern edge.

● Walk about 600 feet and look to the right to see the Isabella Stewart Gardner Museum. After a lifetime of travel and collecting art, Gardner created this Venetian palazzo to house her art collection and gave it to the city in 1903.

Like the Museum of Fine Arts, this collection is too big to fully explore in a day. Gardner had exceptional, if eclectic, tastes (and the money to indulge them); in this collection, works by Rembrandt, Titian, and Botticelli are featured side by side with more homegrown works from John Singer Sargent, who painted a portrait of Gardner herself. If art is less to your liking, or the weather is being unkind, duck into the central covered courtyard, where careful gardening keeps flowers in bloom throughout the year.

● From the museum, retrace your steps to the paths along the Muddy River and turn right.

● After one block, the path swings north again, and you turn right onto Museum Rd. to return to your starting point.

POINTS OF INTEREST

Museum of Fine Arts 465 Huntington Ave., Boston, MA 02115, 617-267-9300

Back Bay Fens Between Fenway and Park Dr., Boston, MA 02115

Fenway Victory Gardens Corner of Boylston St. and Park Dr., Boston, MA 02115, 617-267-6650

Isabella Stewart Gardner Museum 280 Fenway, Boston, MA 02115, 617-566-1401

route summary

1. Begin at the MFA T Station on Huntington Ave. and cross Huntington to enter the Museum of Fine Arts.

2. Exit the museum through the bookstore door and turn right on Museum Rd.

3. Cross Fenway to reach the Back Bay Fens, then turn right on the path to go around the Fens counterclockwise.

4. Turn left on Boylston St. to cross a bridge and then make an immediate left to reenter the Back Bay Fens.

5. Walk straight through the Victory Gardens and return to the path along Park Dr.

6. From the Kelleher Rose Garden, take the path west toward the tennis courts, and then bear left on the path between the track and the river.

7. Turn left on Fenway to return along a path following the southern edge of Muddy River.

8. Turn right on Museum Rd. to return to the starting point at the MFA T Station.

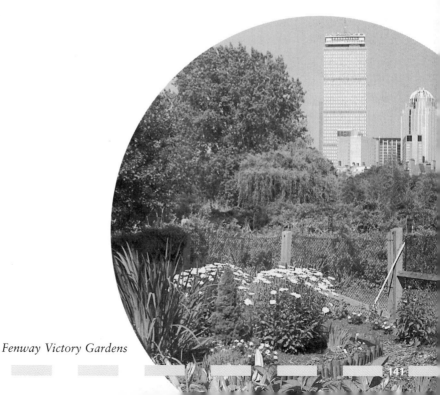

Fenway Victory Gardens

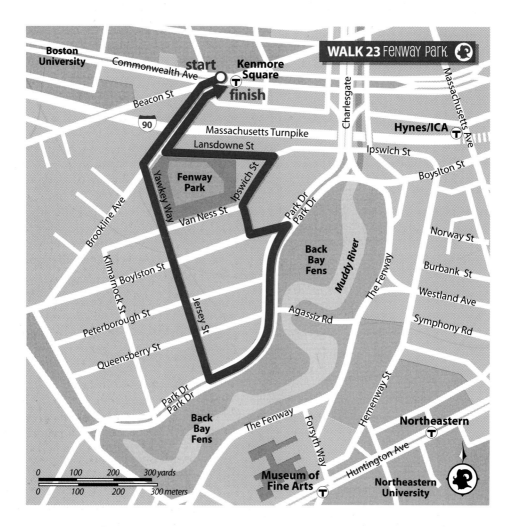

WALK 23 FENWAY PARK

Boston University

Commonwealth Ave

start

Kenmore Square

finish

Beacon St

90

Charlesgate

Hynes/ICA

Massachusetts Ave

Massachusetts Turnpike

Lansdowne St

Ipswich St

Boylston St

Fenway Park

Ipswich St

Yawkey Way

Van Ness St

Park Dr
Park Dr

Norway St

Brookline Ave

Back Bay Fens

Muddy River

Burbank St

Westland Ave

Symphony Rd

The Fenway

Kilmarnock St

Boylston St

Jersey St

Agassiz Rd

Peterborough St

Queensberry St

Park Dr
Park Dr

Back Bay Fens

The Fenway

Forsyth Way

Hemenway St

Northeastern

Huntington Ave

Museum of Fine Arts

Northeastern University

0   100   200   300 yards
0   100   200   300 meters

23 FENWAY PARK: THE LYRIC LITTLE BANDBOX

BOUNDARIES: **Beacon St., Brookline Ave., Park Dr.**
DISTANCE: **Approx. 1¼ miles**
DIFFICULTY: **Easy**
PARKING: **There are several paid parking lots around Fenway Park.**
PUBLIC TRANSIT: **Kenmore Square T Station on the Green Line; busses 8, 55, 57, 60, and 65**

Boston's literary and cultural history may be rich, but for many Bostonians, the real historical treasure of this town is the Red Sox, whose baseball stadium just so happens to be the oldest one in America. Indeed, the history of Fenway Park and the Red Sox is the stuff of legends: Babe Ruth's "curse," Ted William's spectacular home run well into the right-field bleachers, the Red Sox 2004 comeback against the Yankees to win the American League Championship en route to their first World Series victory in nearly a century. It's a magical place. New Englander and writer John Updike perhaps gets Fenway Park the best in the opening of his story about seeing Ted Williams' last game at Fenway, calling it "a lyric little bandbox of a ballpark," offering "a compromise between Man's Euclidean determinations and Nature's beguiling irregularities."

October is the best time to take this tour—especially if it's an October when the Red Sox are still playing. And an October when the Red Sox beat the Yankees en route to another World Series title is the best—if you (and the Sox) can manage it.

● **Begin at the Kenmore Square T Station. As you ascend the stairs, notice the huge Barnes & Noble store on the opposite side of Kenmore Square. Then look up to see the equally large Citgo sign atop the B&N—it is well known to players and spectators alike, as it looms over the famous left-field wall, affectionately called the "Green Monster."**

Although Kenmore Square has seen a lot of changes, it has remained a bustling, vibrant place for much of the past 100 years. In the 1930s through the 1950s, Kenmore Square was a hotspot for jazz, centered around the bar Storyville (in the basement of what was once the Buckminster Hotel and is now Pizzeria Uno, at the corner of Brookline Ave. and Commonwealth Ave.). Another legendary club

was the Rathskeller (better known as simply "the Rat"), which hosted such acts as the Cars, the Dead Kennedys, the Dropkick Murphys, Joan Jett, the Police, the Ramones, R.E.M, Talking Heads, Sonic Youth, and Tom Petty—many before they were famous. The Rat eventually fell victim to urban renewal and now the elite Hotel Commonwealth stands on the site.

● Face Kenmore Square and turn left to walk west on Commonwealth Ave., and then make an immediate left onto Brookline Ave. If it's a game day, this direction may be your only option, as hordes of fans spill out from the T station and head to the ballpark; trying to going anywhere else would be like swimming upstream. On Brookline, you will cross the bridge over Interstate 90 and begin a pilgrimage through a carnival of T-shirt and hotdog vendors, people looking for tickets, people looking to sell tickets, and people looking to sell a variety of other things, both legal and illegal. Students from Berklee College of Music come here to play for a few bucks for beer. Most importantly, you can pick up a copy of the unofficial Sox program, *Boston Baseball*, written by and for the fans—cheaper and more honest than the official Red Sox program.

BACK STORY: AD OR ICON?

The original "Cities Service" sign was erected in 1940 and has undergone numerous renovations and replacements since then, including a high-tech makeover in 2005. Citgo wanted to dismantle the sign in 1983, but the public was so upset by the idea, that the company relit the sign (it had been turned off in 1979 to conserve energy), and it has been glowing brightly at night ever since. The current incarnation is a 60-by-60-foot sign illuminated by thousands of LEDs.

If you want to watch the game from a bar so close you can almost taste the Fenway franks, try the Cask'n Flagon (62 Brookline) or Boston Beer Works (61 Brookline). The Cask'n Flagon is a Fenway Park icon—started in 1969 as Oliver's and changed to Cask'n Flagon a few years later, this little bar with its distinctive gold and green awnings has been serving beer to Sox fans and visitors for years. Boston Beer Works is an award-winning microbrewery, just down Brookline from Cask'n Flagon, and it offers a slightly more updated experience, featuring a rotating menu of more than 50 different styles of beer with whimsical names like Bambino Ale and Victory Red (in honor of the 2004 Red Sox championships) that celebrate Fenway Park and the Red Sox. Try the Kölsch beer, made from an 800-year-old recipe from Cologne, Germany.

- If you survive Brookline, turn left on Yawkey Way to reach the heart of "Red Sox Nation." Named after former Red Sox owner Tom Yawkey, this street becomes part of Fenway Park during games—meaning that on game days you need a ticket to enter this swirling mass of people in Red Sox and anti-Yankee gear. Poke your head into the Souvenir Shop on the right (19 Yawkey Way). Better known as "Twins Souvenirs" or even just "Twins," the store is owned by Twins Enterprises, the company formed by the D'Angelo twins, Arthur and Henry. The D'Angelo brothers got their start selling newspapers in Dorchester when the only English they knew was "two cents paper, mister." Their souvenir shop is now probably the most profitable one in the state. On some days, the line just to get inside stretches out of the store and around the block.

- If you've managed to score tickets, turn left to enter Fenway. With a legendary 37-foot-high, left-field wall called the "Green Monster," a hand-operated scoreboard, a foul line pole named "the Pesky Pole" (after Red Sox player Johnny Pesky), and an irregular shape to accommodate surrounding streets, Fenway Park offers a one-of-a-kind experience. Built in 1912, this stadium has had more than its share of heart-breaks—and (especially after the team's World Series wins in 2004 and 2007) elation. Throughout the season, you can sign up for a tour ($12 for adults) of the stadium and hear its storied history—such as Ted Williams' monster home run in 1946, when he hit the ball some 502 feet away from home plate. His amazing feat is commemo-rated by the red-painted seat 21 in section 42, row 37, where the ball landed in the right-field bleachers. At the time, the man in the seat, Joe Boucher, was unable to catch the ball. After it bounced off his straw hat, the ball disappeared, and Boucher had to go home empty-handed, later declaring, "After it hit my head, I was no longer interested."

- After the game, or on nongame days, continue south on Yawkey Way toward the corner of Yawkey and Van Ness St. Note the banners hanging from the brick of Fenway Park listing the years the Sox have won the World Series. They start in 1903, continue through the teens, when the team was an athletic dynasty, and then there's nothing for 86 years—until the 2004 and 2007 victories. At the corner of Yawkey and Van Ness is the players' entrance, frequently crowded with hangers-on and paparazzi. You can also check out the statue of Ted Williams.

  Continue on Yawkey, past Boylston St., where Yawkey becomes Jersey St. Stop in at the Brown Sugar Cafe, at 129 Jersey. This hole-in-the-wall Thai restaurant has an impressively diverse menu featuring scores of rice dishes, noodles, hot pots, fresh rolls, and a shrimp curry served on a coconut shell.

  From the restaurant, continue south along Jersey St. toward the Back Bay Fens.

- Turn left on Park Dr. and head north to Boylston St., which comes in from the left.

- Cross Boylston and turn left on it to walk a half block to Ipswich St.

- Turn right on Ipswich and follow it north. Fenway Park is directly ahead. When Ipswich reaches Fenway (on Van Ness), follow the street right around the south corner of the park.

- Make a sharp left on Lansdowne St. Although it runs just behind the outfield, Lansdowne, which has undergone some redevelopment in recent years, is almost as famous for its club scene as Fenway is for its baseball. Legendary nightspots like the Boston Tea Party, Metro, 15 Lansdowne, Avalon, and Axis once hosted national acts like Bob Dylan and Van Morrison and homegrown talent like the Receiving End of Sirens.

  For daytime pursuits, try mingling with the crowds gathering outside Gate C on game days. It's the best place to grab a sausage from the carts outside and listen to the crowds from the Green Monster and bleachers seats cheer for the Sox.

If you're lucky, a homer may just land in front of you (be sure to duck, though, especially if you're wearing a straw hat).

● Turn right on Brookline Ave. to return to the Kenmore Square T Station.

POINTS OF INTEREST

Cask'n Flagon 62 Brookline Ave., Boston, MA 02215, 617-536-4840

Boston Beer Works 61 Brookline Ave., Boston, MA 02215, 617-536-2337

Souvenir Shop 19 Yawkey Way, Boston, MA 02215, 617-426-8686

Fenway Park 4 Yawkey Way, Boston, MA 02215, 877-733-7699

Brown Sugar Cafe 129 Jersey St., Boston, MA 02215, 617-266-2928

route summary

1. Begin at the Kenmore Square T Station and walk west on Commonwealth Ave.
2. Turn left on Brookline Ave.
3. Turn left on Yawkey Way, which becomes Jersey St.
4. Turn left on Park Dr.
5. Turn left on Boylston St.
6. Turn right on Ipswich St.
7. Turn left on Lansdowne St.
8. Turn right on Brookline Ave. to return to the Kenmore Square T Station.

Fenway Park scoreboard

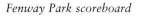

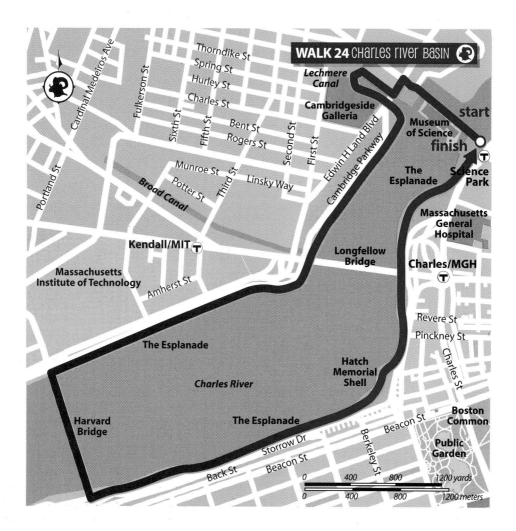

WALK 24 CHARLES RIVER BASIN

Thorndike St
Spring St
Hurley St
Charles St
Fulkerson St
Cardinal Medeiros Ave

Lechmere Canal
Cambridgeside Galleria

start

Museum of Science

finish

Sixth St
Fifth St
Bent St
Rogers St
Second St
First St
Edwin H Land Blvd
Cambridge Parkway

The Esplanade

Science Park

Portland St
Munroe St
Potter St
Third St
Linsky Way
Broad Canal

Massachusetts General Hospital

Kendall/MIT

Massachusetts Institute of Technology

Amherst St

Longfellow Bridge

Charles/MGH

Revere St
Pinckney St
Charles St

The Esplanade

Hatch Memorial Shell

Charles River

Harvard Bridge

The Esplanade

Storrow Dr
Back St
Beacon St
Berkeley St
Beacon St

Boston Common

Public Garden

0   400   800   1200 yards
0   400   800   1200 meters

24 CHARLES RIVER BASIN: SCIENCE, SAILING, AND THE BOSTON POPS

BOUNDARIES: **Monsignor O'Brien Hwy., Cambridge Pkwy., Massachusetts Ave., Storrow Dr.**
DISTANCE: **Approx. 4 miles**
DIFFICULTY: **Easy**
PARKING: **There is a garage at the Museum of Science, and a small, three-hour parking lot off of Charles St. at the Blossom St. Bridge.**
PUBLIC TRANSIT: **Science Park T Station on the Green Line; bus EZ22**

The Charles River divides Boston from its smarty-pants cousin Cambridge, to the north. This walk bridges that gap and features some of the best of both sides. Beginning in Boston's West End, the walk follows greenway on both banks to get you close to the water and never far from lovely views of the city, interesting shopping, and myriad outdoor recreational opportunities.

This is very much a walk for a summer day, when hundreds of small sailboats ply the blue waters of the basin and the parks are full of people enjoying the sunshine.

● Begin at the Science Park T Station at the corner of Charles St. and Monsignor O'Brien Hwy. and follow the pedestrian walk northwest to the Museum of Science. Don't let the T. rex at the door scare you off. The museum is well worth the stop. First opened in 1951, the museum boasts a five-story Imax theater, the world's largest lightning bolt generator, a virtual fish tank, dinosaurs, birds, hands-on activities, and, oddly enough, a Friday night happy hour for adults.

● Once you've sated your inner child (or the one next to you), turn left out of the front entrance (continuing northwest) and make your way past the lines of parked Boston Duck Tour vehicles along the busy and loud O'Brien Hwy. If you haven't done the Duck Tours, you may want to get in line. These immensely entertaining city tours (while not as good as walking) are led by colorful characters with large personalities (everything from a police officer to a superhero) who drive retrofitted World War II amphibious vehicles.

- Turn left on the sidewalks just before Edwin H. Land Blvd.

- At the stairs on the left, just before the Lechmere Canal Bridge, descend to the canal and turn right to walk along the northern edge of the canal. This small water inlet is popular with families paddling along in rented outrigger canoes and tourists snapping pictures from the deck of a water ferry.

  Continue to the end of the canal, and, if you need a break, stop into the Cambridgeside Galleria Mall; bathrooms and a food court are inside on the right.

- From the mall, continue along the path that leads back out to the Charles River Basin along the southern edge of the Lechmere Canal.

- Back at the Charles River, follow the path as it bears right along the water. Stroll to the Charlesgate Yacht Club, one of the Boston area's most exclusive places to park your yacht. Admire the boats for what they are worth (a lot!), and then continue your circumnavigation of the Charles River Basin.

  Along this side of the river, you'll see families fishing the river for striped bass and also get an unparalleled view

Back Story: 364 Smoots and an Ear

In 1958, MIT student Oliver Smoots was laid end to end repeatedly to measure the length of the Harvard Bridge. Because he was, at 5′ 7″, the shortest member of his fraternity pledge class, he was chosen as the unit of measurement in this fraternity initiation activity. The bridge is equal to 364 Oliver Smoots—plus an ear. You can count them off yourself in 10-smoot increments on the bridge. When the bridge was rebuilt in 1990, the state agreed to retain the Smoot measurements.

of Beacon Hill rising from the river like some sort of ancient city. The gold dome of the State House is just visible past the brownstones.

About halfway between the Museum of Science and the Longfellow Bridge (described by tour guides and tour bus drivers as the "salt-and-pepper-shaker bridge," for its pillars) is a public dock—the perfect vantage point for taking pictures and enjoying the sun. As you continue down the path along the water, MIT will be visible on the right, with its famous Great Dome looming above Killian Court. You may also be inspired to take a quick detour in Killian Court at MIT to check out the various sculptures in the courtyard, which include *La Grande Voile* ("the Big Sail") by Alexander Calder.

● Continue along the canal to Massachusetts Ave., and then turn left to take the Harvard Bridge back over the Charles River. Sometimes called the Mass. Ave. Bridge by the same folks who came up with "the salt-and-pepper-shaker bridge," this bridge was built in 1891 and named after the Cambridge college it led to at the time (MIT would move to Cambridge more than 20 years later, in 1916). As you cross, guess how many "smoots" it takes to cross the bridge (hint: read the "Back Story").

● Once back on the Boston side, take the ramp back down to the water's edge and turn left to walk east along the embankment through the Charles River Esplanade. In 1910, this area was developed as a public park shortly after the construction of the Charles River Dam; it was expanded in 1928.

● At Storrow Lagoon, take the footbridge on the left to the narrow spit of land separating the Charles River from the lagoon. This land was added in 1949 to make up for park land lost to the construction of Storrow Dr., which cuts right along the edge of the esplanade. The added land created the Storrow Lagoon (which will be on your right as you walk) and offers great views of the Charles River and the Cambridge side (on the left).

● Walk east along the waterside as far as you can on the spit of land and take the last bridge back to the mainland. The path will bring you right up to the Hatch Memorial Shell, site of Boston's internationally famous Fourth of July Boston Pops concert and fireworks show. The first Boston Pops concert was conducted by Arthur Fielder in 1929, and although many of the classics like the *1812 Overture* have remained, the Fourth of July concert now includes a dramatic fireworks show and a TV/webcast that attracts millions.

Continue along the shore. Just before the Longfellow Bridge are the Community Boating docks, America's oldest public sailing club and where many Bostonians learn to sail. A little bit farther are the Teddy Ebersol Red Sox Fields at Lederman Park. Named in memory of a young Red Sox fan, these poorly drained fields near the river were repaired to form a wonderful community resource after a coalition of nonprofit groups raised nearly $2 million.

● At the end of the path, cut across the parking lot by the tennis courts to save walking an uninspiring section of Charles St. At Monsignor O'Brien Hwy., turn right and use the crosswalks to return to the Science Park T Station.

POINTS OF INTEREST

Museum of Science 1 Science Park, Boston, MA 02114, 617-723-2500

Boston Duck Tours 3 Copley Pl. (main office), Boston, MA 02116, 617-267-DUCK

Cambridgeside Galleria Mall 100 Cambridgeside Pl., Cambridge, MA 02141, 617-621-8666

Hatch Memorial Shell On the Esplanade, Boston, MA 02114, 617-727-1300

Community Boating 21 David Mugar Way, Boston, MA 02114, 617-523-1038

ROUTE SUMMARY

1. Begin at the Science Park T Station and follow the pedestrian walk northwest.
2. Turn left on the sidewalk just before Edward H. Land Blvd.
3. Turn left to descend the stairs just before the Lechmere Canal Bridge.
4. At the bottom of the stairs, turn right to follow the path along the northern edge of the canal.
5. From the mall, continue along the path to return to the river along the southern edge of the canal.

6. At the river, turn right to follow the path as far as the Harvard Bridge.

7. Turn left to cross the Harvard Bridge.

8. At the end of the bridge, turn left and take the ramp down to the footpath along the river, and turn left.

9. Turn left at the first path to get on the spit of land in between the lagoon and the river.

10. Return to the mainland using the northernmost bridge and continue north on the waterside path.

11. Cut through the parking lot with the tennis courts to Monsignor O'Brien Hwy. and turn right to return to the Science Park T Station.

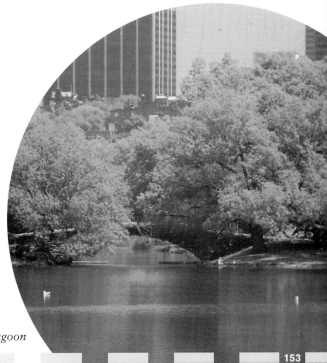

Storrow Lagoon

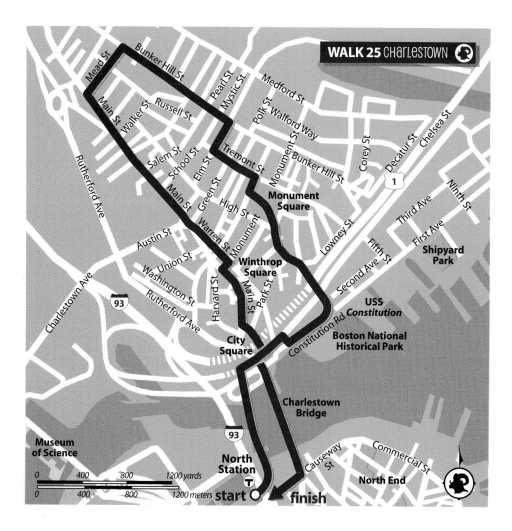

WALK 25 CHARLESTOWN

Mead St
Bunker Hill St
Main St
Walker St
Russell St
Pearl St
Mystic St
Medford St
Polk St
Walford Way
Salem St
School St
Elm St
Green St
Tremont St
Monument St
Bunker Hill St
Corey St
Decatur St
Chelsea St
1
Ninth St
Monument Square
Main St
High St
Monument
Lowney St
Third Ave
First Ave
Fifth St
Shipyard Park
Austin St
Warren St
Winthrop Square
Rutherford Ave
Union St
Washington St
Rutherford Ave
Harvard St
Main St
Park St
Second Ave
USS Constitution
Constitution Rd
Boston National Historical Park
Charlestown Ave
93
City Square
Charlestown Bridge
Museum of Science
93
North Station
Causeway St
Commercial St
North End

0 400 800 1200 yards
0 400 800 1200 meters

start   finish

25 CHARLESTOWN: TWO HILLS AND THE TRUTH

BOUNDARIES: **Causeway St., Main St., Mead St., Bunker Hill St., Constitution Rd.**
DISTANCE: **Approx. 3¼ miles**
DIFFICULTY: **Moderate**
PARKING: **There is paid parking at the TD Banknorth Garden on Causeway St. and the Boston National Historic Park on Constitution Rd.**
PUBLIC TRANSIT: **North Station T Station on the Green and Orange lines; busses 92, 93, 111, 325, 326, 353, 354, 355, 424, and 426**

When the English settlers first arrived in Massachusetts in 1629, they set up camp in Charlestown, favoring its sloped hills and ocean views. They couldn't locate any freshwater on the peninsula, however, and soon moved across the water to found the city of Boston. Later, in 1775, Charlestown's historical legacy was cemented, when a ragtag group of volunteer soldiers inflicted some serious damage on the army of the British Empire.

This walk should be done in late spring—June 17, to be exact. It was on that day American farmers, merchants, and part-time soldiers stood up to the mighty British Army in what has become erroneously known as the Battle of Bunker Hill (see "A Tale of Two Hills" on page 157). The Colonial Army lost the hill by the end of the day, but the British Redcoats paid dearly for it. Go celebrate with the annual costumed reenactment and festivities.

● **Begin at the North Station T Station and follow Causeway St. north to Portal Park, on the left.**

● **Turn left to go through the park, then bear right to follow the paths to the north side, where you should look for the blue HARBORWALK signs marking the walkway toward the Charles River Locks (note that the Harborwalk also continues along the water toward the North End). Completed in 1978, the locks and dam regulate the water level in the Charles River Basin and provide passageway for boats. However, there is also a fish ladder and the area attracts lots of folks with fishing rods. If you don't have a taste for fish, bang on the bells made by local artist Paul Matisse to make your own songs.**

- At the end of the locks, continue north through Paul Revere Park, one of Boston's newest parks. It was the first of the new parks associated with the Big Dig project and is a great place for flying kites and running dogs.

- From the park, turn right on the pathway that leads under Rte. 99. After the underpass, this becomes Constitution Rd.—follow it toward the Boston National Historical Park. Before heading to the big ships, stop at the Bunker Hill Pavilion at 55 Constitution Rd. The center, one stop on the Freedom Trail, is a good place to go to the bathroom, get something to drink, and brush up on your Revolutionary War history with a multi-media presentation called "The Whites of Their Eyes."

From the pavilion, move on to the Boston National Historical Park at the Charlestown Navy Yard. The park was formed in 1974 when the Charlestown Navy Yard was closed after nearly 175 years of building and servicing warships (it was one of six warship-building naval yards in the country). Today, the park is home to the USS *Constitution* ("Old Ironsides"), the oldest commissioned warship in the world (it launched in 1797), and the USS *Cassin Young*, a World War II destroyer, as well as historic buildings, water shuttles to other parts of Boston Harbor, and a variety of exhibits on maritime history. The *Constitution* is open for tours almost every day (barring some federal holidays). On the Fourth of July, the old ship is towed into the harbor and brought back into its berth in the opposite direction to even out the weathering. The *Cassin Young*, which was retired in 1960, is typical of the type of destroyer-class ships built at the yard, and it can also be toured on most days. While at the Navy Yard, you may want to check out the Constitution Museum (separate from the actual ship), the 1805 Federal-style commandant's house, the ropewalks where rope was made, and the barracks for the sailors.

- From the park, return to Constitution Rd. and follow it north to the pedestrian underpass below Rte. 1.

- Cross under Rte. 1 to join Chestnut St. and follow Chestnut north to Adams St.

- Turn left on Adams and follow it to Winthrop Square, a former colonial militia training grounds.

Back Story: a Tale of Two Hills

In June of 1775, the British Army in Boston was ticked off. A few months earlier, they had been soundly beaten back to the barracks by the Minute Men of Lexington and Concord, and now the Colonial Army had gathered around Boston. Learning of an imminent attack by the Redcoats, the Colonial Army decided to build a fortification on Bunker Hill in Charlestown to make their stand.

But instead of setting up on Bunker Hill on the night of June 16, the Patriots quickly dug in fortifications on Breed's Hill, about a quarter mile away. Israel Putnam, a second brigadier general of the forces from Connecticut, decided that Breed's Hill was a better choice because it was close enough for their cannons to reach the British forces as they attacked. However, because of the last-minute switch, it became known as the "Battle of Bunker Hill," even though it was fought on Breed's Hill.

It was a brutal battle (as most are), and although the British ended the day occupying the hill, they sustained more than twice as many casualties as the colonists, and this severely hurt the British forces in New England. A monument to Dr. Joseph Warren, a revolutionary patriot and leader, was erected on the site in 1794, with the cornerstone of the obelisk laid on the 50th anniversary of the battle in 1825. The monument was completed in 1843 and dedicated on June 17 of that year.

● From Winthrop Square, walk north up the hill on Winthrop St. to Monument Square and the Bunker Hill Monument. The grey granite obelisk is an impressive beacon. Climb the 294 steps to the top for a unique view of Boston and the surrounding neighborhoods (including the real Bunker Hill just 2,000 feet to the northwest). For a primer on the history of this battleground and why you shouldn't call it Bunker Hill, go into the visitor lodge (open daily except major holidays). There is no fee, but the monument is open only between 9 AM and 5 PM.

● Exit the park on the west side and turn right on Monument Square.

- At the northern edge of the square, turn left. What was Monument Square (the Bunker Hill Monument is surrounded on all sides by the street called "Monument Square") becomes Bartlett St. as you move west.

- Turn right on Elm St.

- Turn left on Bunker Hill St. As you begin to trudge up the hill, you'll catch a glimpse of the steeple of the Church of Saint Francis DeSales Parish. The church stands atop the real Bunker Hill.

- Just past the Church of Saint Francis DeSales Parish, turn left on Mead St. and continue to its end at a set of stairs. Stop for a moment on the stairs to take in the view across Charlestown, the Zakim Bridge, and, if it's clear, Boston just beyond. Note how the towers of the bridge resemble the Bunker Hill Monument.

- Descend the stairs and continue along Mead St.

- Turn left on Main St. and continue to Thompson Square.

- At Thompson Square, bear left to join Warren St.

- Turn right on Pleasant St. and celebrate your own conquering of Charlestown with a beer at the Warren Tavern, at 2 Pleasant St. Serving up suds since the colonial days, this tavern was reputed to be one of Paul Revere's favorite watering holes.

- Turn left on Main St. At 55–62 Main St. is the John Larkin House (a private home today, so please respect the current owners' property). Although his original house was destroyed in the Battle of Bunker Hill, this Federal-style home once belonged to Deacon Larkin, who provided Paul Revere with his horse for Revere's famous midnight ride to warn of the Redcoats' march on Lexington and Concord. Revere is famed for shouting, "The British are coming! The British are coming!" while riding through the suburbs of Boston. But the history is notoriously incorrect here; more likely, Revere was muttering some four-letter words about the British. After all, the Redcoats did capture him (he was later released). Nonetheless, Revere made it to Lexington before he was captured, and he does deserve credit for rousing the Minute Men of Lexington and Concord. The next day was the famous "shot heard 'round the world"—the first exchange of gunfire in the Revolutionary War—at the Northern Bridge in Concord.

Continue on Main St. as it winds through a lovely little neighborhood before reaching City Square, a rectangular park at the corner of Rte. 99 (New Rutherford Ave.) and Chelsea St. City Square is the site the Massachusetts Bay Company chose in 1629 to start their new colony. Unfortunately, there was no freshwater in the area, and the colonists relocated across the bay on the Shawmut Peninsula. The foundation of what is believed to be early colonist John Winthrop's 1630 house were found here. For more information, read the interpretive displays near the fountain and sculptures at the center of the park. If you are feeling hungry, try the Mediterranean cuisine at Olives, 10 City Square, celebrity chef Todd English's home kitchen.

● Walk diagonally south through the park, use the crosswalk to cross Chelsea St., and then head south across the Charlestown Bridge on New Rutherford Ave. From the bridge, you'll have a great view of both the Charles River Locks below and the Leonard P. Zakim Bunker Hill Bridge, the widest cable-stayed bridge in the world. Zakim was a local activist and hero who worked tirelessly for the youth of Boston and for cancer patients until his own death by cancer in 1999.

● On the other side of the bridge, turn right on Causeway St. to return to the North Station T Station.

POINTS OF INTEREST

Boston National Historical Park Charlestown Navy Yard, Charlestown, MA 02129, 617-242-5601

Bunker Hill Pavilion 55 Constitution Rd., Charlestown, MA 02129, 617-241-7575

USS *Constitution* Charlestown Navy Yard, Charlestown, MA 02129, 617-242-7511

USS *Cassin Young* Charlestown Navy Yard, Charlestown, MA 02129, 617-242-5644

Bunker Hill Monument Monument Square, Charlestown, MA 02129, 617-242-5641

Warren Tavern 2 Pleasant St., Charlestown, MA 02129, 617-241-8142

Olives 10 City Square, Charlestown, MA 02129, 617-242-1999

route summary

1. Begin at the North Station T Station and follow Causeway St. north to Portal Park.

2. Turn left to enter park, and then bear right to follow the paths to the north end of the park.

3. Follow the HARBORWALK signs through the Charles River Locks.

4. At the end of the locks, continue north through Paul Revere Park.

5. At the end of the park, turn right on the path that leads under Rte. 99. This path becomes Constitution Rd., which you follow to the Boston National Historical Park.

6. From the park, return to Constitution Rd., and follow Constitution to the pedestrian underpass under Rte. 1.

7. Cross under Rte. 1 to join Chestnut St. and head north on Chestnut.

8. Turn left on Adams St. and follow it to Winthrop Square.

9. From Winthrop Square, walk north on Winthrop St. and up the steps to the Bunker Hill Monument.

10. Exit the park on the west side and turn right on Monument Square.

11. Turn left on Bartlett St.

12. Turn right on Elm St.

13. Turn left on Bunker Hill St.

14. Turn left on Mead St. and descend the stairs at the end of Mead.

15. At the bottom of the stairs, continue straight ahead on Mead.

16. Turn left on Main St.

17. At Thompson Square, bear left to join Warren St.

18. Turn right on Pleasant St.

19. Turn left on Main St.

20. Cross to the southern side of City Square, cross Chelsea St., and then head south across the Charlestown Bridge.

21. Once across the bridge, turn right on Causeway St. to return to the North Station T Station.

*Winthrop St. leading to the
Bunker Hill Monument in Charlestown*

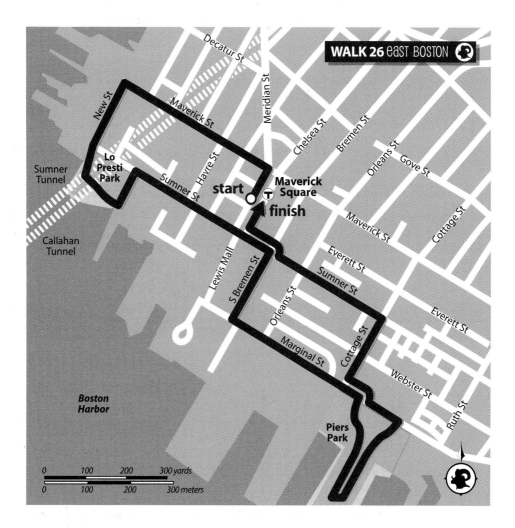

WALK 26 east BOSTON

Decatur St

New St

Maverick St

Meridian St

Chelsea St

Bremen St

Orleans St

Gove St

Sumner Tunnel

Lo Presti Park

Havre St

Sumner St

start

Maverick Square

finish

Maverick St

Cottage St

Callahan Tunnel

Lewis Mall

S Bremen St

Everett St

Sumner St

Everett St

Orleans St

Marginal St

Cottage St

Webster St

Boston Harbor

Piers Park

Ruth St

| 0 | 100 | 200 | 300 yards |
| 0 | 100 | 200 | 300 meters |

26 east BOSTON: a former cattle ranch takes off

BOUNDARIES: Maverick St., Cottage St., Marginal St., New St.
DISTANCE: Approx. 2 miles
DIFFICULTY: Easy
PARKING: There is free, two-hour parking in Maverick Square and at Piers Park.
PUBLIC TRANSIT: Maverick Square T Station on the Blue Line; busses 114, 116, 117, 120, and 121

Once the home of shipbuilders, merchants, and a cattle ranch, East Boston is now a wonderfully vibrant, multi-ethnic community. (It's also the site of Boston's Logan International Airport.) This area saw difficult times in the 1980s and '90s, but recently it has received significant interest and investment. This walk circles East Boston's Maverick Square, sampling the best of the neighborhood, from an eco-oriented affordable housing project to a lovely waterfront park on a reclaimed pier.

This is not a walk for winter, as East Boston gets a strong, cold wind off Boston Harbor. However, once warmer weather arrives and spring flowers begin to open, this route beckons those on foot for a stroll along the water, where you'll get unbeatable views of downtown Boston.

● **Begin at the Maverick Square T Station. This area was once a 500-acre cattle ranch owned by Samuel Maverick, whose name is attached to this square as well as a number of surrounding buildings. East Boston's proximity to Boston as well as the ocean has made it an attractive location for shipbuilders, and, particularly after the airport was built, waves of immigrants. Canadians came first, then Irish, followed by Russians and other Eastern Europeans. In the 20th century, Italians and South Americans (particularly Brazilians) have made East Boston home.**

From the T station, head north along Maverick Square, toward the corner of Meridian and Maverick streets. On the left, at 40 Maverick Square, is the green-and-white awning of La Sultana, a Mexican bakery with a loyal following. Devotees swear by the *arepas* (Colombian quesadillas) and or the *rolla de fresa* (strawberry jelly roll).

You can grab a little something here or at the multi-ethnic Bella's Market (73–75 Maverick Square), and bring it to a lovely park just around the corner on Maverick St. Continue up Maverick Square to view the Neoclassical Sovereign Bank, with its elegant dome and gray columns, on the northwest corner of the square.

● Turn left on to Maverick St. and walk two blocks to the park across from the Church of the Most Holy Redeemer. This huge Gothic Revival church was built in 1857 and has remained intensely popular among the many immigrant groups in the area. Across the street from the church is a small park with curving paths that fan out from a central fountain, making the park look like a pinwheel from above.

● Once Maverick St. dead-ends, turn left on New St. and follow it all the way to the water. On your left is the far edge of Maverick Landing, one of the most successful housing developments in the city. In 1942, Boston Housing Authority built this "war housing," then called Maverick Gardens, with 414 affordable units for veterans and other white Bostonians. The first families of color moved in during the mid-1960s, followed eventually by groups from Latin America, Somalia, and Bosnia.

By 2000, the sense of community among these disparate groups was very strong, and Maverick Gardens had one of the lowest crime rates of any of the Boston Housing Authority properties. Unfortunately, the infrastructure was not as strong, and the buildings began to fall into disrepair. A private developer completely razed the complex and replaced it with a mix of 426 affordable and market-rate apartments. The new buildings include green-building features such as solar panels, fiberglass windows for insulation, and a cogeneration unit to provide energy.

● At the point where New St. meets Sumner St., leave New and continue heading south across the plaza to Harborwalk along the water. Take a moment to look out across the water, then turn left and follow Harborwalk to Lo Presti Park.

● Walk east through this 4-acre park, and enjoy the views. On the left is an open green for games and picnicking. On the other side of Sumner St. are Maverick Landing's bright and cheery brick façades, with their solar panels soaring above the roofline. Across the water to your right, you can see Boston's skyline.

Just before the path bends to the left to return to Sumner St., take a moment to read the Harborwalk interpretive marker describing the history of Carlton Wharf. A local merchant named John Carlton built the wharf in 1851, and although the wharf fell on tough times, it is slated for a new housing complex.

On the other side of Carlton Wharf is the site of the Hodge Boiler Works, famous only for making the boiler used in the 1951 movie *African Queen*. This area is also slated for renewal; projects already underway include a 116-unit condominium with a cafe, a bed and breakfast, and a marina.

- Turn right on Sumner St. If you're hungry, visit popular Taqueria Cancun, at 192 Sumner, on the left side.

- Turn right on S. Bremen St. and follow it for one block to Marginal St., which turns off to the right.

- Instead of turning right, take the path on the left that skirts the East Boston Greenway and then joins the other end of Marginal St. The East Boston Greenway is a reclaimed railroad and trolley track that is now a 3-mile corridor for biking, walking, jogging, and in-line skating. The 40-ton blue caboose was donated by Conrail to commemorate the greenway's history as a railroad track.

- On the other side of the greenway, continue east on Marginal St. to Piers Park, about one block on the right. The 6.5-acre park is Massport's $17 million gift to East Boston in exchange for Logan Airport (which occupies the other major chunk of East Boston). Developed with significant community input, the park offers

Piers Park

grassy areas, playgrounds, an amphitheater, public bathrooms, and absolutely stunning views of Boston.

- Enter the park from the north and walk south toward the water. As you enter the park, look to your right to see the site of a future project at Piers Park. It has not been developed yet but will hopefully expand the park with additional facilities. Directly ahead is the Piers Park Sailing Center, offering inexpensive sailing lessons; its adaptive sailing program for people with disabilities is particularly impressive, but the whole center deserves praise for its mission of getting people out on the water.

- Once at the water's edge, make your way southeast along the path and then head out on the long pier stretching into the Boston Harbor. Part of Piers Park, this pier is a great place for a stroll along the water, and the two pavilions in the middle offer a glimpse into the history and cultural heritage of East Boston. The walls of the first pavilion are inscribed with a number of designs and patterns reflecting the area's many immigrant groups, while the second is dedicated to Donald McKay, a ship-builder who made East Boston one of the preeminent shipyards of the mid-19th century by producing some of the fastest clipper ships in the world. His ship, *The Flying Cloud*, broke the speed record for a trip around Cape Horn. From the McKay Pavilion, downtown Boston looks close enough to reach out and touch. Looking back toward land, you can also get great views east to Logan Airport and north to the old merchants' homes and what is called the "Golden Stairs"—an actual staircase often used in the mid-19th century by smugglers hauling goods up from the waterfront to merchants at the top of the hill.

- Return to the base of the pier, and take the path bearing right to walk by the parking lot and then loop back to the snack shack and bathrooms, before exiting the park at the intersection of Marginal St. and Cottage St.

- Head north on Cottage St., passing the Ciampa Community Garden on the right, where early spring daffodils can brighten even the greyest of days.

- Turn left on Sumner St.

- Turn right on Maverick Square to return to your starting point.

POINTS OF INTEREST

La Sultana 40 Maverick Square, East Boston, MA 02128, 617-568-9999

Bella's Market 73–75 Maverick Square, East Boston, MA 02128, 617-567-7152

Taqueria Cancun 192 Sumner St., East Boston, MA 02128, 617-567-4449

Piers Park Sailing Center 95 Marginal Rd., East Boston, MA 02128, 617-561-6677

ROUTE SUMMARY

1. Begin at the Maverick Square T Station and walk north on Maverick Square.
2. Turn left on Maverick St.
3. Turn left on New St. and continue south toward the water after the intersection of New and Sumner streets.
4. Turn left on Harborwalk and follow it to the end of Lo Presti Park.
5. Turn right on Sumner St.
6. Turn right on S. Bremen St. and walk to Marginal St., which comes in from the right.
7. Turn left on the walking path to skirt the bottom of the East Boston Greenway and then continue east by following Marginal St.
8. Take the first path on the right to enter Piers Park and walk south toward the water.
9. At the shoreline, walk southeast toward the pier.
10. Walk down the pier and then retrace your steps and walk to the circular fountain at the base of the pier.
11. From the base of the pier, take the path bearing right to walk by the parking lot and then to the snack shack and bathrooms.
12. Exit the park at the intersection of Marginal and Cottage streets and head north on Cottage.
13. Turn left on Sumner St.
14. Turn right on Maverick Square to return to your starting point.

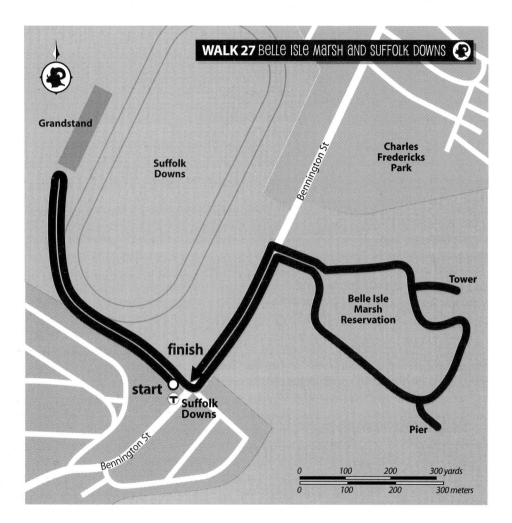

WALK 27 BeLLe ISLe MarSH and SUFFOLK DOWNS

Grandstand

Suffolk Downs

Bennington St

Charles Fredericks Park

Tower

Belle Isle Marsh Reservation

finish

start

Ⓣ Suffolk Downs

Bennington St

Pier

| 0 | 100 | 200 | 300 yards |
| 0 | 100 | 200 | 300 meters |

27 Belle Isle Marsh and Suffolk Downs: Things That Fly

BOUNDARIES: **Waldemar Ave., Bennington St., Belle Isle Park**
DISTANCE: **Approx. 2 miles**
DIFFICULTY: **Easy**
PARKING: **There is free parking at Bell Isle Marsh.**
PUBLIC TRANSIT: **Suffolk Downs T Station on the Blue Line; busses 119 and 120**

This walk starts at Suffolk Downs (where trainer Tom Smith discovered the famous racehorse Seabiscuit) and then explores lovely Belle Isle Marsh with views of Winthrop Island and Logan Airport. The paths are clear and easy to follow, so this tour makes a wonderful, easy stroll if you are looking for a bit of nature in East Boston.

Spring brings flowers, nesting birds, and occasionally even warm sunshine. Try this walk on a Sunday afternoon, when families bring their kids, or early on a weekday morning when it is still and quiet.

● **Begin at the Suffolk Downs T Station. Exit the station through the back door and go down the stairs to where the Suffolk Downs shuttle busses come. Go through the gate directly across the street and follow the access road around the southern edge of the track and around the main entrance.**

Suffolk Downs opened in 1935, mere months after gambling had been legalized in Massachusetts. It was here, in 1936, that famed horse trainer Tom Smith first laid eyes on the horse that became one of America's favorite sports figures, Seabiscuit. After winning numerous races across the country, Seabiscuit and Smith returned to Suffolk Downs in 1937 to win the Massachusetts Handicap, the most prestigious race held at the track each year. Today, Suffolk Downs is the only remaining thoroughbred racetrack in New England, with live races that run May through mid-November. The track is open all year for race simulcasts from other tracks around the world.

- If it's not a racing day, you can enter the grandstands through the main entrance and wander around inside of one of America's most storied racetracks.

- From the grandstands, retrace your steps along the access road to the Suffolk Downs T Station and walk through the station to the exit on Bennington St.

- Turn left on Bennington St. and walk to the main entrance of the Belle Isle Marsh Reservation on the right.

- Turn right to walk down the access road, and then bear right into the parking lot. You'll find a map here that covers the park's 28 acres of trails and fields. This 152-acre park is just part of the 241-acre Belle Isle Marsh, Boston's last remaining salt marsh. Salt marshes are formed in low-lying areas near the ocean where fresh- and saltwater mix. In addition to providing flood control during storm surges, these marshes serve as important habitat for a variety of animals and plants, some of which are specially adapted to adjust to the differences that occur as the tide surges in and out. Not surprisingly, human development along coastlines have simultaneously destroyed many salt marshes while increasing their importance.

- From the parking lot, walk to the right and take the southernmost trail. It leads straight ahead to wooden walkway jutting out over the grasses and swampland toward the water. Although the trail around the marsh is gravel, it can get a little muddy in wet weather so bring good shoes.

  As you walk, keep your ears tuned for the sounds of birds and keep your eyes peeled for field mice, voles, and garter snakes darting (or slithering) across the paths. In addition to the chirping of crickets, the sounds of songbirds, and the swaying of grasses in the wind, you may, depending on wind and approach patterns, hear the thunderous roar of a jet. Don't worry, it won't land on you; Logan Airport is less than a mile to the south.

- Follow the path to the wooden walkway sticking 140 feet out into the marsh. It provides an excellent viewpoint for spying muskrats, snapping turtles, and herons in the waters. From here, you can also see the town of Winthrop and Logan Airport.

- Return to the main path and turn right to continue on your counterclockwise tour of Belle Isle. The path heads north before swinging around to the left along an artificial channel.

- Turn right to go over the bridge and to the lookout tower. If you happen to be here on a day when the jets are landing in this direction, wait about five minutes for a thrill. Large airplanes, coming in from around the world, appear suddenly over the crest of the little neighborhood of Beachmont, and drop even lower before screaming by and landing at Logan.

- From the tower, retrace your steps back across the small bridge to the main path and turn right on the path that shoots north before swinging west for a quiet amble along a small waterway and hitting the access road.

- Retrace your steps out the access road and turn left on Bennington St. to return to the Suffolk Downs T Station.

POINTS OF INTEREST

Suffolk Downs 111 Waldemar Ave., East Boston, MA 02128, 617-567-3900

Belle Isle Marsh Reservation Bennington St. (across from Suffolk Downs), East Boston, MA 02128, 617-727-5350

ROUTE SUMMARY

1. From the Suffolk Downs T Station, exit through the back door, cross the driveway, enter the gate, and follow the access road to Suffolk Downs.
2. Retrace your steps and walk through the T station to exit onto Bennington St.
3. Turn left on Bennington St. to walk to the Belle Isle Marsh Reservation.
4. Turn right on the access road and walk to the southernmost trail that begins in the parking lot.
5. Follow the path to its end and then continue along the wooden pier jutting over the marsh.

6. Retrace your steps from the pier to the main path and turn right to follow the path around the waterside.

7. Turn right to cross the bridge and walk to the tower.

8. Retrace your steps from the tower to the main path and turn right to follow the path to the access road.

9. Retrace your steps on the access road and turn left on Bennington St. to return to the Suffolk Downs T Station.

*The neighborhood of Beechmont,
just north of Belle Isle Marsh*

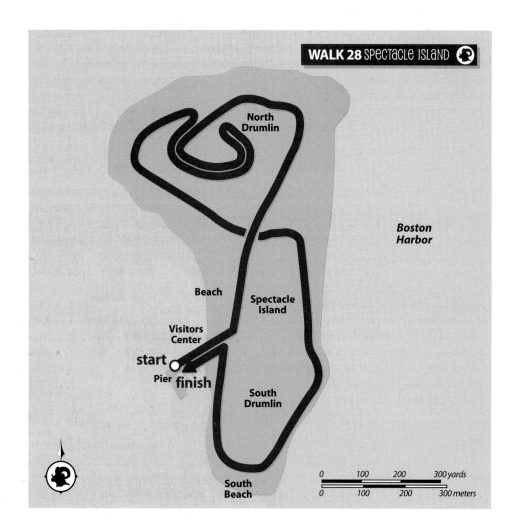

WALK 28 SPECTACLE ISLAND

North
Drumlin

Boston
Harbor

Beach

Spectacle
Island

Visitors
Center

start

Pier finish

South
Drumlin

South
Beach

| 0 | 100 | 200 | 300 yards |
| 0 | 100 | 200 | 300 meters |

28 Spectacle Island: a Closer Look at One of the Harbor Islands

BOUNDARIES: **Boston Harbor, Long Wharf**
DISTANCE: **5 miles**
DIFFICULTY: **Moderate with some hills**
PARKING: **There is paid parking near each of the ferry departure points.**
PUBLIC TRANSIT: **Take the ferry from Long Wharf, EDIC Pier, Hull at Pemberton Point, or Quincy at Fore River Shipyard. For more information about getting to the Boston Harbor Islands, visit www.bostonislands.org.**

One of Boston's greatest gems is its collection of 34 small islands scattered throughout the harbor. Many of these outcroppings provided excellent protection for the harbor, and you can still visit forts—some crumbling and some well-preserved—that dot the harbor. Some of the islands have also been used for less savory purposes—for garbage dumps, sources for timber, and factories for rendering dead horses.

However, with great investment from the city of Boston and the Department of Conservation and Recreation, 17 of these islands have been cleaned up and maintained as parks with walking trails, visitors centers, interpretive displays, and campgrounds. One of the best choices for a short trip is the 121-acre Spectacle Island, accessible by ferry from Long Wharf. During the Big Dig project, Spectacle received more than 3.7 million cubic yards of dirt—that's 4,400 barge loads over five years. The dirt was used to completely reshape and expand the island, making it into a wonderful place to walk, with unbelievable views of Boston. In addition to the well-maintained paths, there is an eco-designed visitors center, a pristine beach, and picnic tables, pavilions, and benches throughout the island.

While this tour is best only during the warmer months (May to October), the high season brings mobs of crowds looking to escape the heat of downtown. Visit in June or September for a sense of solitude, the promise of clear weather, and enough sunshine for leisurely picnicking.

- Start at Boston's Long Wharf (call 617-223-8666 for a current ferry schedule). The boat trip to Spectacle Island takes just 15 minutes and provides lovely views of the Boston waterfront, Logan Airport, and Castle Island.

- From the boat dock, follow the pier up to the visitors center to get your bearings, use the bathroom, buy a snack, pick up a map and guide to the island, and view the exhibits dedicated to the island's history. You can also relax in one of the white Adirondack chairs on the front porch or read up on the green technology employed on the islands. Spectacle Island is striving to be a "zero-emission" park, with extensive use of renewable energy sources and water conservation. For example, there are solar panels on the roof of the visitors center to help power all the electric vehicles used on the island.

- From the visitors center, take the path leading directly north toward the northern rise of the island (called the "North Drumlin"). When colonists arrived in the area, Spectacle Island consisted of two rises connected by a thin isthmus, making it look like a pair of spectacles, which gave rise to the name of the island. The Native Americans used the island for hunting and fishing until the colonists stripped the land of its timber and used it to graze cattle during the early 18th century. Since then, the island has been home to a variety of different things, including two tourist hotels, a quarantine hospital, a factory for making glue, and a garbage dump. The city of Boston stopped bringing its trash here in 1957, and in 1992, started bringing in dirt from the Big Dig to cap the landfill and create a new island shape. It now looks a bit more like a mallet with a wide northern tip and a skinnier southern "handle."

  As you head up the hill toward the North Drumlin, look to the left, where four granite pillars rise from the water along West Beach. Now the home of cormorants, these pillars mark the dock of Nahum Ward's Rendering Factory, which transformed dead horses into glue, hides, and Neat's Foot Oil (a leather softener) in the late 1800s. Take a breath of the clean, salty air and be glad those days are over.

- At the first junction, take the path that bears right (north) to circle around the eastern edge of the North Drumlin. At the junction, there is an interesting signpost describing how the topography of Spectacle Island has changed over the years. If you're ready to take a rest, you can walk east on a short path to a shade pavilion by the water, where you can watch the sailboats scoot by. Beyond the pavilion is Long Island, which the city uses for a number of social service programs for the homeless, a navigational marker for Logan Airport, an abandoned missile base, and the remains of an organic farm. Unlike most of the other islands in the bay, Long Island is closed to the public.

Continue walking toward the northeast side of the North Drumlin to go around counterclockwise. As you round the base of North Drumlin on your way to its summit, you'll be rewarded with views of large tankers plying the water of the harbor; Deer Island, with its distinctive white wastewater treatment tanks; Logan Airport; and, finally, Boston, just 4.5 miles away across Dorchester Bay. From here, Boston's landmarks are crystal clear: From left to right (south to north), look for the Prudential and Hancock towers in Back Bay, the Federal Reserve Building marking the start of the Financial District, Fort Independence guarding the entrance to Boston Harbor, the Harbor Towers of downtown, and the very top of the Leonard P. Zakim Bunker Hill Bridge crossing over to Charlestown.

Although it is tempting to stop here at the viewing station, you've got a summit to reach. Keep following the path counterclockwise around the drumlin until you reach a wide, open picnicking spot with another shade pavilion and four or five picnic tables spread across the lawn. The views from up here are even better than from the path below. In addition to the earlier landmarks across Dorchester Bay, you can look to the east to Long Island, south to Moon Island, and to the west to see Thompson Island.

● Leave the summit on the same path you ascended earlier. As you curve

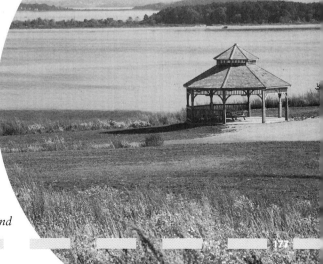

Shade pavilion on Spectacle Island

around to the north (going clockwise now), you come to a juncture on the north side of the North Drumlin.

● Take a sharp left (west) at this juncture, and then walk 300 feet to the next Y junction.

● Take the lower (closer to the water) of the two paths that branch out to curve around the western edge of the drumlin. Here you get great views to the west of Thompson Island, once a thriving trading outpost and now home to an Outward Bound facility. To the south, you can see the pier where you arrived and the visitors center, with photovoltaic panels on the roof.

Follow the path around to the saddle linking the two drumlins, and be on the lookout for fields of shrubs with pretty white flowers. These are "false spirea," just one of the 28,000 varieties of shrubs and grasses planted on the island after the dirt was dumped over the landfill. All of the plants were chosen for their ability to thrive in the harsh conditions on the island, and many are native to Spectacle. The path will lead you back to a juncture near the island's center.

● Turn left at this junction and walk 150 feet north on the path you were on earlier.

● At the next juncture, you will be facing due east with a shade pavilion directly in front of you; turn right (south) here to cross to the eastern side of the island, and walk 400 feet to a Y junction.

● Bear left on the path that is closest to the water to circle around the South Drumlin in a clockwise direction. This brings you down along the South Beach, where sea glass and, occasionally, Native American artifacts can be discovered. From some of the artifacts found on the island, scientists guess that the island may have been used as far back as 8000 years.

As you circle the island's southernmost point, enjoy the unfettered views to the south to the bridge connecting Moon and Long islands, and to Quincy Bay beyond.

Follow the trail north to return you to the visitors center and the pier. Be sure you have checked the ferry schedule and make it back before the final trip back into Boston.

POINT OF INTEREST

Boston Harbor Islands National Recreation Area 617-223-8666

route summary

1.   From the visitors center, follow the path leading north toward the North Drumlin.

2.   At the first juncture, bear right to take the eastern path that leads around the eastern side of the North Drumlin.

3.   Continue on the path to ascend the North Drumlin counterclockwise.

4.   From the summit, retrace your steps clockwise to the first juncture on the north side of the North Drumlin.

5.   Turn sharp (west) at the first juncture and walk 300 feet.

6.   At the Y junction, take the right (closer to the water) path that leads around western edge of the North Drumlin.

7.   At the juncture near the center of the island, turn left and walk 150 feet north to a junction near a shade pavilion.

8.   Turn right (east) to access the shore path, and follow this south toward the South Beach.

9.   At the next juncture (after 400 feet), bear left to take the path closer to the water, and follow this around the southern tip of the island to return to the visitors center.

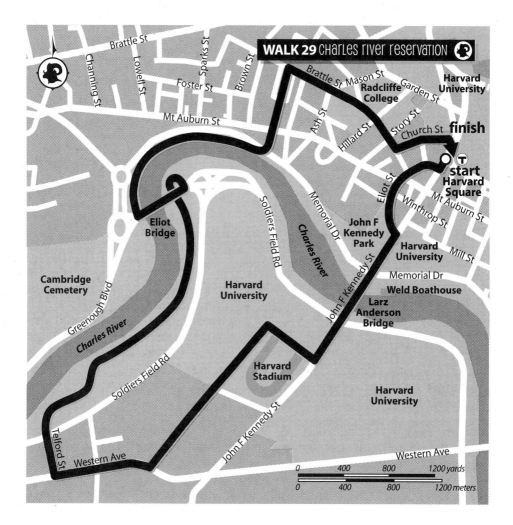

WALK 29 charles river reservation

Brattle St
Channing St
Lowell St
Sparks St
Brown St
Foster St
Mt Auburn St
Brattle St
Mason St
Radcliffe College
Garden St
Story St
Church St
Harvard University
finish
Ash St
Hillard St
Eliot St
start
Harvard Square
Mt Auburn St
Winthrop St
Mill St
Eliot Bridge
Soldiers Field Rd
Memorial Dr
Charles River
John F Kennedy Park
John F Kennedy St
Harvard University
Memorial Dr
Weld Boathouse
Larz Anderson Bridge
Cambridge Cemetery
Greenough Blvd
Charles River
Harvard University
Soldiers Field Rd
Harvard Stadium
John F Kennedy St
Harvard University
Telford St
Western Ave
Western Ave

| 0 | 400 | 800 | 1200 yards |
| 0 | 400 | 800 | 1200 meters |

29 Charles river reservation: riparian rambles

BOUNDARIES: **Greenough Blvd., Memorial Dr., N. Harvard St., Western Ave.**
DISTANCE: **Approx. 3½ miles**
DIFFICULTY: **Easy**
PARKING: **There is a free public parking lot on Soldiers Field Rd., across from Everett St.**
PUBLIC TRANSIT: **Harvard Square T Station on the Red Line; busses 8 and 66**

This section of the Charles is less crowded and less showy than the Esplanade and the Charles River Basin near the Museum of Science, but it's also more relaxing and peaceful. Perhaps because of that, this area attracts strolling lovers, sunbathing students, and river-watchers who indulge in quiet contemplation on benches along the banks. Also keep an eye out for crew teams from the local schools knifing through the water.

This is a lovely walk for spring, when the sun coaxes blooms out of the trees, crew teams onto the waters, lovers onto the paths, and sun-worshippers to the grassy fields. Though it is a long walk (and can be extended east or west along the 17 miles of parkland comprising the Charles River Reservation), it is perfectly flat, uses paved paths, and has plenty of benches for resting.

- Begin at the Harvard Square T Station and walk west on Brattle St. to Brattle Square. On the western edge of Brattle Square, just past where Brattle St. cuts off to the right, look for *DooDoo* (not what you think). It is a bronze statue of beloved Brattle Square puppeteer Igor Fokin's favorite character, a little, alien-like creature with big ears sticking out from the sides of his head, eyes on top, and a long, bugle nose. When Fokin died in 1996, his friends and family erected this tiny, 10-inch shiny bronze statue. It stands right on the very edge, near the road.

- Walk south on Brattle Square, which becomes Eliot St. and bears off to the left.

- Turn right on John F. Kennedy St. to head south toward the Charles River. On the right, just before the intersection between JFK and Memorial Dr., is the John F. Kennedy Park. Pause for a moment to read the inscription on the granite pillars of the two park entrances; they feature some of JFK's most inspirational passages from his speeches. The park, a pleasant, 5-acre spot by the river, is populated by students and businesspeople taking a lunch break. Be warned against walking barefoot here; the oaks and elms lining Memorial Dr. drop acorns and sticks that make the grass treacherous. The upside is that the park is planted with indigenous plants and flowers that bloom in May, around Kennedy's birthday.

Continue on JFK St. across the Larz Anderson Bridge and stop for a moment to watch the crew teams go by. If you're on this walk during the third full weekend in October, you may be sharing your perch with thousands of college kids gathering for the annual Head of the Charles Regatta—the largest two-day rowing event in the world. Many of the 55 different regatta races begin by the Boston University Boathouse downstream and end just past the Eliot Bridge after a grueling 3-mile row. The Harvard University Boathouse is on the left as you start over the bridge.

● On the other side of the bridge, use the crosswalks to cross to the southwest corner of Soldiers Field Rd. and N. Harvard St. Walk through the gate on your right into the Harvard University athletic campus, and bear left to head south along the path parallel to N. Harvard St.

● Just past the Murr Center (indoor tennis courts), turn right on the walkway to cut along the north end of Harvard Stadium, America's oldest collegiate football stadium. Built in 1903 from a design based on a stadium in Athens, Greece, it has hosted thousands of football games, lacrosse games, Olympic soccer games, rock concerts, ice hockey games, political rallies, and, for two years, New England Patriots football games.

● When you arrive at the Gordon Indoor Track, turn left to walk between the football stadium and Harvard's baseball field, and then angle across the baseball fields of the William E. Smith Playground to the southwest corner, near Western Ave.

● Turn right on Western Ave. to walk west toward Telford St.

● Turn right on Telford St.

● Cross Soldiers Field Rd. using the pedestrian bridge and enter the parking lot. If you have an interest in theater, you may want to check out the outdoor stage at the Publick Theatre, which is set on an artificial island in the middle of an artificial lagoon.

On summer nights, you can see a mix of professional and aspiring actors in plays from the likes of Tom Stoppard, Anton Chekhov, and, of course, William Shakespeare.

● From the theater, face the river and turn right to head northwest on the paths along the water. The Charles River Basin is managed by the Department of Conservation, with help from the nonprofit Charles River Conservancy (CRC). The CRC works on a number of education and capital projects, including a new skate park and making the Charles "swimmable" again. The paths along both sides of the Charles are well maintained and popular with joggers, bikers, and walkers. In addition, the evenly spaced benches provide lovely vantage points to watch the activity on the water. As you work your way along the Boston side of the river, there will be a number of path options, and any one is fine, as long as you keep the river on the left.

● At the Eliot Bridge, cross under the bridge and then make a sharp right turn to loop back around and cross the Charles using the sidewalk on the north side of the bridge. Eliot Bridge is named after Charles Eliot, who bought up much of the land for and helped design the Charles River Basin in 1893.

● Once over the bridge, turn right to follow the paths that lead past the red boathouse for Buckingham Browne and Nichols (a local private school) on the right. You will then walk through a parking lot in front of the Cambridge Boat Club and rejoin the walking path by the water on the Cambridge side of the Charles. Between the Eliot Bridge and the Larz Anderson Bridge is one of the prettiest sections of the Charles; in spring, cherry blossoms line the paths and the light shimmers on the water in the late afternoon.

Longfellow House

- When the Charles River begins to bend around again to the south, look for a small park on the other side of Memorial Dr., and turn left to cross Memorial and walk north through the park.

- Cross Mt. Auburn St. and continue north through the granite pillars with the black iron gates into Longfellow Park. From here, follow the rectangular expanse of grass leading to the Longfellow Memorial at the far end. Next, take the stairs behind the memorial to another swatch of green leading to the Longfellow House, at 105 Brattle St.

  A close friend of Ralph Waldo Emerson, Charles Dickens, and Nathaniel Hawthorne, Henry Wadsworth Longfellow was an institution unto himself at Harvard, where he taught from 1836 to 1854. After retiring from Harvard he devoted himself full time to writing and lived in this bright yellow home with the black shutters and white pillars for nearly 40 years, until his death in 1882. The house is now a National Historic Site and run by the National Park Service; tours are available on Wednesdays through Sundays, from May through October.

- After exiting the Longfellow House, walk east (left when facing the street) on Brattle St., which was once known as "Tory Row" because of its residents' wealth and loyalty to the crown. Much of the street's original architecture has been carefully preserved. Keep your eye out for widow's walks, painted chimneys, and ornamental fences.

  As Brattle bends around before reentering the Harvard Square area, note the big boxy building on the right. This is the home of the American Repertory Theatre, one of the nation's finest acting companies. Serving up an eclectic blend of contemporary plays and reimagined classics, it is well worth stopping in for tickets.

- Turn left on Church St. Just past the parking lot on your left is one of the better ice cream places in Cambridge. Look for the lounging cow sign, and duck into Lizzy's Ice Cream, at 29 Church, for a treat before continuing on Church.

- Turn right on Massachusetts Ave. to return to the Harvard Square T Station.

POINTS OF INTErEST

John F. Kennedy Park Memorial Dr., Cambridge, MA 02167, 617-727-5250

Harvard Stadium 95 N. Harvard St., Allston, MA 02134, 617-495-2211

Publick Theatre 1175A Soldiers Field Rd., Brighton, MA 02135, 617-782-5425

Longfellow House 105 Brattle St., Cambridge, MA 02138, 617-876-4491

American Repertory Theatre 64 Brattle St., Cambridge, MA 02138, 617-547-8300

Lizzy's Ice Cream 29 Church St., Cambridge, MA 02138, 617-354-2911

rOUTE SUMMArY

1. Begin at the Harvard Square T Station and follow Brattle St. west to Brattle Square.
2. From Brattle Square, take Eliot St. south.
3. Turn left on John F. Kennedy St. and head south to cross the Larz Anderson Bridge over the Charles River.
4. Cross to the southwest corner of Soldiers Field Rd. and N. Harvard St., then walk through the gates on the right to Harvard's athletic campus and bear left on the path to parallel N. Harvard.
5. Turn right just past the Murr Center to cut along the north end of Harvard Stadium.
6. At Gordon Indoor Track and Tennis Facility, turn left to walk between the football stadium and Harvard's baseball field, and then angle across the William E. Smith Playground to the southwest corner along Western Ave.
7. Turn right on Western Ave.
8. Turn right on Telford St.
9. Cross Soldiers Field Rd. on the pedestrian bridge and walk along the western edge of the parking lot to the paths along the Charles River.
10. Face the water and turn right to follow paths to the Eliot Bridge.
11. Cross under the bridge and make a sharp right to loop around and cross the Charles on the Eliot Bridge.
12. After the bridge, turn right to follow the paths along the Charles again.
13. Just after the river's northernmost point, turn left to cross over Memorial Dr. and walk north through the small park.
14. Exit the park and cross Mt. Auburn St., to enter Longfellow Park and walk north.
15. Turn right on Brattle St.
16. Turn left on Church St.
17. Turn right on Massachusetts Ave. to return to the Harvard Square T Station.

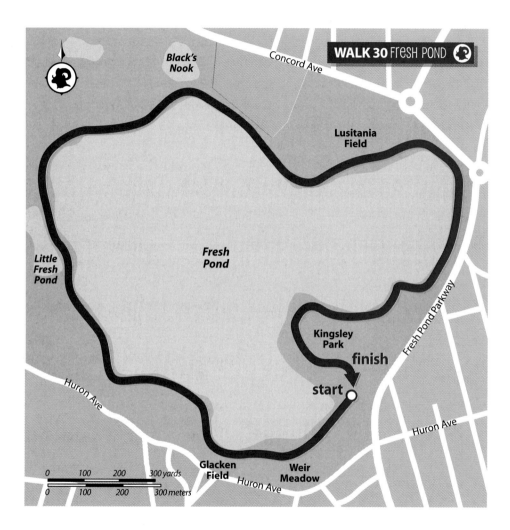

WALK 30 FRESH POND

Black's Nook

Concord Ave

Lusitania Field

Little Fresh Pond

Fresh Pond

Kingsley Park

Fresh Pond Parkway

finish

start

Huron Ave

Glacken Field

Weir Meadow

Huron Ave

Huron Ave

0   100   200   300 yards
0   100   200   300 meters

30 FreSH POND: COUNTING THe BIrDS

BOUNDARIES: **Fresh Pond Pkwy., Concord Ave., Blanchard Rd., Grove St., Huron Ave.**
DISTANCE: **2½ miles**
DIFFICULTY: **Easy**
PARKING: **There is resident parking only at the reservation, and limited street parking on Huron Ave. and Concord Ave.**
PUBLIC TRANSIT: **Busses 72, 74, 75, and 78**

Two hundred thirty. That's how many birds have been identified in the Fresh Pond Reservation since 1984. This whopping number includes 11 species listed as endangered, threatened, or of special concern by the Massachusetts Division of Fisheries and Wildlife. It also includes the 13 different species of ducks (like the ring-necked, ruddy, and canvasback) and 35 different species that nest at the lake in the spring. This "kettle lake," formed in a depression left by a glacier, anchors the North Cambridge area and offers many opportunities for running, walking, biking, golf, and, not surprisingly, bird-watching. As a result of the diversity of people Fresh Pond attracts, you'll catch plenty of different languages as you walk.

Although the paths may be a little muddy after it rains, go to Fresh Pond in the springtime when everything is in bloom and the birds are migrating. If you feel like migrating a bit farther yourself, it's possible to extend this walk by connecting with any number of nearby intercity bike paths. Note: Fresh Pond is still an important part of Cambridge's drinking water supply, so observe all regulations.

●   **Begin at the Kingsley Park parking lot, off Rte. 2 (Fresh Pond Pkwy.), and turn left on the path to go around the pond clockwise. The Fresh Pond Reservation includes the 155-acre Fresh Pond and 162 acres of surrounding land. The pond has been used as fishing waters, an ice supply, a place to dig clay for bricks, and a water reservoir. Although it's no longer used for industrial purposes, the pond still delivers water to Cambridge (purified at the Walter J. Sullivan Water Purification Facility, which you will pass on this walk). The primary use, though, is for recreation, and the area is often packed with walkers, runners, and players of all sorts.**

The first place you come to is Weir Meadow, an open space great for picnicking. The name of the meadow, "weir," means "small dam," referring to the dam that used to run across the stream here. Fresh Pond and the surrounding streams once were teeming with fish, and the Native Americans, as well as the settlers who came later, built weirs to trap fish.

- Continue past the meadow to Glacken Field. At the far end of Glacken Field is the Golf Course Clubhouse, accessible by a trail up through the woods on your left. In addition to snacks and drinks, there are public bathrooms just inside the doors on the right. Glacken Field is a popular recreation area, and includes a tot lot closer to the road. On the Glacken Slope (between Glacken Field and Fresh Pond), there is a hardwood forest favored by many of the migratory song birds that come to the area in the spring. If you look closely, you might find a yellow warbler or a song sparrow hidden among the branches.

- From Glacken Field, continue along the western edge of Fresh Pond to Little Fresh Pond, popular with kids who like to catch frogs and dogs that . . . well, just like water.

- Continue your walk around the northern edge of Fresh Pond to another small pond, Black's Nook. Once a part of Fresh Pond, Black's Nook is now a separate body of water. Those who are interested in looking for songbirds and amphibians who make their home here should follow a small path that runs west and northwest around the lake.

- Pass Black's Nook and walk to Sousa's Rock and Neville Place, an assisted-living community and site of a soccer field, butterfly meadow, and community gardens. Look for the large stand of American beech trees on the bank below the Neville Manor building.

- Continue east on the trail, which winds past Lusitania Field. Wildflower fans should take a quick detour to the meadow just west of Lusitania Field to check for Queen Anne's lace, chicory, thistle, and white avens. This is another great place to spy songbirds.

- At Fresh Pond Pkwy., follow the road south toward the Walter J. Sullivan Water Purification Facility. Although this seems like a strange place to find art, the water purification facility actually has two interesting permanent art installations (as well as some public bathrooms). The first is Michele Turre's painted satellite map of the city's reservoir system on the second floor. There is also an installation of pipes, landscaping, bronze, and real water, entitled *Drawn Water*. A 2,500-square-foot map inlaid on the floor of the entry hall shows the underground pipes, water fountains, swimming pools, and ponds of the city, which includes the winding blue streak of the Charles River. The map blends elements inside and outside, including landscaping, pipes, the water intake, and a drinking fountain that arcs water. And there's more even farther afield; throughout Cambridge, there are 13 bronzed utility covers with unique water images. To help you find these treasures, the map on the floor of the lobby shows the locations of each one. The entire installation was done by Mags Harries and Lajos Heder in 2001.

● From the water purification facility, continue south to Kingsley Park, and take the trail on the right to walk out along the water before returning to your car or the bus stop.

POINTS OF INTEREST

Kingsley Park Fresh Pond Pkwy., Cambridge, MA 02138, 617-349-4793

Walter J. Sullivan Water Purification Facility
250 Fresh Pond Pkwy., Cambridge, MA 02138, 617-349-6489

ROUTE SUMMARY

1. Begin at Kingsley Park parking lot and turn left to follow the path clockwise around Fresh Pond.

Fresh Pond

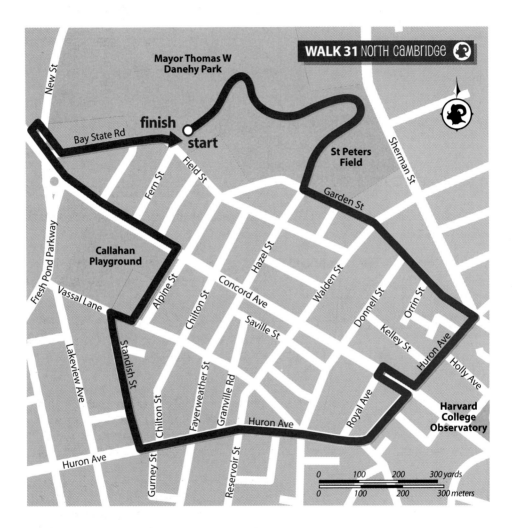

WALK 31 NORTH CAMBRIDGE

Mayor Thomas W Danehy Park

New St

finish

start

Bay State Rd

St Peters Field

Sherman St

Field St

Fern St

Garden St

Callahan Playground

Hazel St

Fresh Pond Parkway

Vassal Lane

Alpine St

Concord Ave

Walden St

Donnell St

Orrin St

Chilton St

Saville St

Kelley St

Huron Ave

Holly Ave

Lakeview Ave

Standish St

Fayerweather St

Granville Rd

Royal Ave

Harvard College Observatory

Huron Ave

Chilton St

Huron Ave

Gurney St

Reservoir St

| 0 | 100 | 200 | 300 yards |
| 0 | 100 | 200 | 300 meters |

31 NorTH Cambridge: a Big Park and PUBLIC art

BOUNDARIES: **Danehy Park, Cambridge Common, Concord Ave.**
DISTANCE: **Approx. 2½ miles**
DIFFICULTY: **Moderate**
PARKING: **There is free public parking at Danehy Park.**
PUBLIC TRANSIT: **Busses 72, 74, 75, and 78**

What many people forget about Cambridge is that along with its intellectual endeavors and undergraduate pranks, this is a workin' town. With its proximity to Boston and the lower cost of living, Cambridge has its share of earnest, hardworking neighborhoods. North Cambridge is one of those, and this tour takes in a green oasis built on a capped landfill, a quiet, tree-lined neighborhood, a campus filled with dedicated students, the thriving Concord Ave., and a shop that is almost literally on fire.

Pick a sunny Saturday during soccer season in the fall, when Danehy Park is alive with young people playing sports and Radcliffe is buzzing with activity. The fall foliage will provide the color and the neighborhoods will provide the charm.

● Start at the parking lot of the Mayor Thomas W. Danehy Park, at the corner of Field St. and Fern St. To build this 50-acre park in 1990, the city placed 1.5 tons of grass and wildflower seed and 18 acres of sod over an existing landfill. Take the path on the left to head north.

● Face the soccer field at the top of the hill, and turn right to skirt the soccer field and make your way (north) over to the southern edge of the football field and track. At that point, you will encounter the main park path (it's wide enough for a car). Cross this path and continue north toward the football field for another 170 feet.

● Turn right at the first junction to ascend the highest point in the park, where you will find Mierle Laderman Ukeles' *Turnaround/Surround* art installation. It consists of two circular spaces for performances, a "glassphalt" path made with 22 tons of crushed glass and mirror, and accompanying landscaping. Cantabrigians (the name of those who live in Cambridge) brought in 10 tons of glass and mirror for the project, and the

Spectrum Glass Company in Washington donated the rest. In winter, when all is buried under snow, this hill becomes Cambridge's premier sledding slope.

● After enjoying the view, retrace your steps down the hill and walk to the main intersection, with the football field behind you, a soccer field to the right, and baseball fields to your left.

● Turn left and follow the path east toward the park's Sherman St. entrance. Look at the ground around the water play area to see John Devaney's *Wheeler Water Garden*, a painted mural of a pond, complete with frogs and lily pads. Also at the Sherman St. entrance are bathrooms and, during limited hours, a snack shack with a lovely mural by Holly Alderman.

● From the mural, take the path that leads due south and skirts the eastern edge of Danehy Park before cutting across Roethlisberger Memorial Park (a softball field will be on the left, with trees and an open space on the right) and ending at Garden St.

● Turn left to walk southeast on Garden St. This section of the walk is through a nice, quiet neighborhood of two- and three-story houses with well-kept yards and, in the spring, flowering trees.

● Turn right on Huron Ave. and follow it three blocks to Concord Ave.

Take time for a snack at the Hi-Rise Bakery, at 208 Concord. With a large, rough, wooden, communal table and fantastic breads, it's the type of place that locals swear by and visitors wish they had in their town.

● For more cerebral fare, turn right on Concord Ave. and take a short jaunt northwest to the Boudreau branch of the Cambridge Public Library (public restrooms here), at 245 Concord Ave. The library is worth seeing just for a peek at the front desk. This colorfully painted piece of furniture, designed by Mitch Ryerson, is made of birch, cherry, and maple wood, and is full of odd shapes and angles, with a carved panel on the front depicting books stacked in front of a Cambridge skyline.

- Retrace your steps to the corner of Huron Ave. and Concord Ave. and turn right (south) on Huron (it's downhill here). This is one of the most pleasant stretches in Cambridge. Dotted with darling local stores and blooming trees, Huron Ave. feels like a village square. One highlight is the Fishmonger, at 252 Huron. Featured in the excellent 2004 indie film *American Wake*, this locally owned fish market is typical of the unique offerings you'll find along Huron. At 361 Huron, you can succumb to your inner child and play with stuffed animals at Henry Bear's Park, a loveable shop with plenty of fans. Also make a point to stop at the Bryn Mawr Bookstore, at the corner of Huron and Standish St. Browse their street-side cupboard and then step inside to make your purchase.

- Turn right on Standish St. and follow it north.

- Turn right on Vassal Ln. and then take an immediate left onto the walkway leading along the eastern edge of a school toward the Callahan Playground.

- Turn left on Concord Ave. and follow it to Adams Fireplace Shop, on the right at 505 Concord Ave. If you have ever put a match to newspaper underneath a pile of kindling in a fireplace, or even just snuggled down on a couch in front of a fire, this store is worth visiting. The dark and narrow shop offers row after row of fireplace "things," from brass irons, to 19th-century French marble-handled fire pokers, to canvas log carriers, to wood pellets.

- Retrace your steps on Concord Ave. to Bay State Rd. and turn left on Bay State (which becomes Field St.) to return to Danehy Park.

POINTS OF INTEREST

Mayor Thomas W. Danehy Park 99 Sherman St., Cambridge, MA 02138, 617-349-4895

Hi-Rise Bakery 208 Concord Ave., Cambridge, MA 02138, 617-876-8766

Cambridge Public Library 245 Concord Ave., Cambridge, MA 02138, 617-349-4017

Fishmonger 252 Huron Ave., Cambridge, MA 02138, 617-661-4834

Henry Bear's Park 361 Huron Ave., Cambridge, MA 02138, 617-547-8424

Bryn Mawr Bookstore 373 Huron Ave., Cambridge, MA 02138, 617-661-1770

Adams Fireplace Shop 505 Concord Ave., Cambridge, MA 02138, 617-547-3100

ROUTE SUMMARY

1. Begin at the parking lot of Mayor Thomas W. Danehy Park, at the corner of Field and Fern streets, and take the path on the left to head north.

2. Facing the soccer field, use the path on the right to skirt the soccer field and continue past the junction with the main park path.

3. At first junction after the main path, turn right to ascend the highest point in the park.

4. Retrace your steps to the intersection with the main park path and turn left to head east toward the Sherman St. entrance.

5. From the *Wheeler Water Garden* mural, head south on the path that skirts the eastern edge of the park and then cuts across Roethlisberger Memorial Park to Garden St.

6. Turn left on Garden St.

7. Turn right on Huron Ave.

8. Turn right on Concord Ave. and walk to the Cambridge Public Library at 245 Concord.

9. Retrace your steps to the corner of Concord and Huron Ave. and turn right on Huron.

10. Turn right on Standish St.

11. Turn right on Vassal Ln. and then take an immediate left on the pathway leading to Callahan Playground.

12. Turn left on Concord Ave. and continue to Adams Fireplace Shop at 505 Concord.

13. Retrace your steps on Concord Ave. and turn left on Bay State Rd. to return to the Danehy Park.

Cambridge Public Library

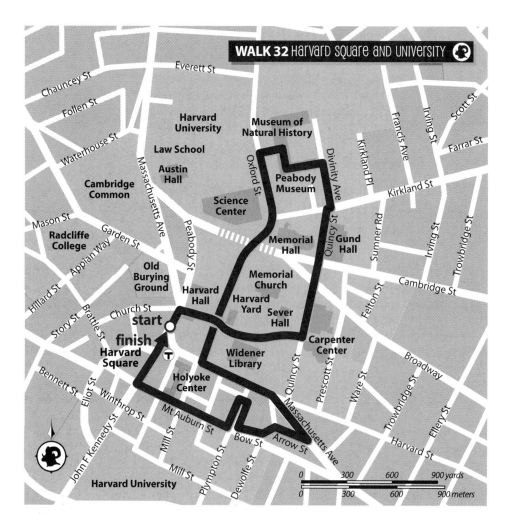

WALK 32 Harvard Square and University

Everett St

Chauncey St

Follen St

Harvard University

Museum of Natural History

Francis Ave

Irving St

Scott St

Waterhouse St

Law School

Austin Hall

Oxford St

Peabody Museum

Divinity Ave

Kirkland Pl

Farrar St

Cambridge Common

Science Center

Kirkland St

Mason St

Garden St

Massachusetts Ave

Peabody St

Memorial Hall

Quincy St

Gund Hall

Sumner Rd

Irving St

Trowbridge St

Radcliffe College

Appian Way

Memorial Church

Hillard St

Story St

Old Burying Ground

Harvard Hall

Harvard Yard

Cambridge St

Brattle St

Church St

start

Widener Library

Felton St

Sever Hall

Carpenter Center

Prescott St

Ware St

Broadway

finish

Harvard Square

Holyoke Center

Quincy St

Massachusetts Ave

Bennett St

Eliot St

Winthrop St

Mt Auburn St

Mill St

Plympton St

Bow St

Arrow St

Harvard St

Trowbridge St

Ellery St

John F Kennedy St

Mill St

Dewolfe St

Harvard University

0   300   600   900 yards

0   300   600   900 meters

32 Harvard Square and University: The Hallowed Halls of Academia

BOUNDARIES: Mt. Auburn St., John F. Kennedy St., Harvard University, Quincy St.
DISTANCE: 2 miles
DIFFICULTY: Easy
PARKING: Paid parking is available on Church St.
PUBLIC TRANSIT: Harvard Square T Station on the Red Line; busses 66, 69, 71, 72, 73, 74, 75, 77, 77A, 78, 86, and 96

Harvard needs no introduction. The school, founded in 1636 on the fields of John Harvard's estate, has become one of the world's preeminent academic institutions, with a long, long list of distinguished alums. And yet, as this walk demonstrates, Harvard University and Harvard Square—that wonderful, bustling hub of activity—remain accessible.

To make this an authentic college campus tour, this walk is best when students are around. Choose a day in early fall when the leafy yards provide cool shade but it's still warm enough to truly enjoy the ice cream at the end.

● Get your bearings at the Out of Town News, at 0 Harvard Square. Converted from an old T station, this venerable institution has been the meeting place for people and the starting point for tours for more than 20 years.

From here, head north on Massachusetts Ave. to Church St. and the First Unitarian Church of Cambridge. It was here, on August 31, 1837, that a young Ralph Waldo Emerson delivered what Oliver Wendell Holmes called America's "Intellectual Declaration of Independence." In essence, Emerson told the assembled graduating Harvard students and their teachers that the European literature they had been studying was old and musty and that they needed to spend their energies on creating a uniquely American literature. The speech helped cement Emerson's growing reputation as a radical thinker and a firebrand—one who would eventually be barred from giving public talks at Harvard.

● From the church, cross Massachusetts Ave. to enter Harvard through the Johnston Gate. Students have been entering Harvard Yard through this area for more than 360 years.

The large brick building on the left is the second edition of Harvard Hall. The first one burned down in 1764, taking with it the majority of the college library at the time. Only one book from John Harvard's original collection survived, saved by a student who had smuggled it out of the library earlier that night. Legend has it that the student, realizing the importance of the last remaining book from John Harvard's collection, brought it to the college president for safekeeping. The president thanked the student and then expelled him for taking a book from the library without permission.

Just past Harvard Hall, also on the left, is Hollis Hall, a residence for first-year students. In addition to transcendentalists like Emerson and Henry David Thoreau, this hall has been home to more contemporary figures like Tommy Lee Jones and Al Gore. Residences like Hollis are not "dorms" as we might think of them; they are considered "colleges" within the university. After living in colleges in or near Harvard Yard during freshman year, students move to one of 12 houses for the remainder of their undergraduate careers. (A 13th house is designed for nonresident students.) Each house has a resident master and a staff of tutors, as well as a dining hall and library, and maintains an active schedule. Student loyalty to their college is often fierce and steadfast and can outlast their loyalty to Harvard itself.

● Stride across Harvard Yard to the statue of John Harvard. Known as the "statue of the three lies," this is not really a statue of John Harvard, who died in 1638 without ever having his portrait taken. Instead, Daniel Chester French used a friend as a model for the sculpture, which was installed in 1884. The second "lie": John Harvard did not found Harvard. It was founded by the Massachusetts Bay Colony, and then named after Harvard, a young minister who died suddenly and left the college his 400-volume library as well as 780 pounds sterling. And, lastly, the date on the statue is wrong. Harvard was founded in 1636, not in 1638.

The building behind the statue is University Hall, designed by Boston architect Charles Bulfinch. It contains the offices of the dean of the faculty of Arts and Sciences and the dean of Harvard College.

- Cut around the south side of University Hall to the great steps of Widener Memorial Library. The library is named for Harry Elkins Widener, who died on the *Titanic* (it's said he went back to his room to get a book and never made it off the ship). The center of the largest academic library system in the world, Widener is where many Harvard students go to study (which means it's a great place for hanging out and not getting any studying done). However, you must be a student to enter the library and browse the 65 miles of bookshelves hidden behind its Corinthian columns, so unless you wear the crimson, you'll have to admire from the outside.

- Standing on the Widener steps with your back to the library, turn right to take the path that slips east between Sever and Emerson halls. Sever Hall, on your left, is a Romanesque-style building designed by architect Henry Hobson Richardson, who also designed Trinity Church in Copley Square, as well as the train station in Newton Centre, among other buildings in Boston.

  Emerson Hall—named, of course, for Ralph Waldo Emerson, who graduated from Harvard in 1821—contains an inscription from Psalm 8:4 above its front columns: "What is man that thou art mindful of him?" Emerson was banned from giving public speeches on the Harvard campus when his find-God-in-nature brand of transcendentalism was deemed too radical for the good Unitarian faculty of Harvard.

  Follow the path between Sever and Emerson to Quincy St.

- At Quincy St., turn left and continue to Kirkland St., crossing Broadway and Cambridge St. along the way. The Fogg Art Museum and the Busch-Reisinger Museum (connected to the Fogg Art Museum

Emerson Hall

by a second-floor passageway), at 32 Quincy, cover Western art from the Middle Ages to the present. The Fogg is noted for its collections of early Renaissance Italian paintings, Impressionist and post-Impressionist works, and early 19th-century French art. The Busch-Reisinger Museum is solely devoted to art from the German-speaking world. Both museums are part of the university and are open during regular business hours Monday through Saturday.

● At Kirkland St., take a short jog right.

● Make an immediate left to continue north on Divinity Ave. Note Divinity Hall on the right, at 14 Divinity Ave. where a young Ralph Waldo Emerson gave one of his two speeches that made him persona non grata at Harvard for almost 30 years.

Continue north on Divinity Ave. to the Peabody Museum of Archaeology and Ethnology, at 11 Divinity. The museum houses an excellent collection of Native American artifacts and is connected to the Harvard Museum of Natural History. You can move from one museum to the other via the third floor, and one ticket gets you into both museums. The Natural History Museum highlights include 3,000 glass models of flowers, the first triceratops ever discovered, and a 1,600-pound amethyst geode.

● Exit the Museum of Natural History through the front door on Oxford St. and turn left to follow Oxford south to Kirkland St.

● At the corner of Oxford and Kirkland, follow the sidewalk that leads around the south side of Harvard's Science Center, across the pedestrian plaza above Cambridge St., and to the north gates of Harvard. On your left, the soaring red brick hall with the striped roof and spires is Memorial Hall, dedicated to the fallen soldiers of the Civil War. It is one of the finest examples in the country of an architectural style called "High Victorian Gothic." Although it looks very much like a cathedral, it is actually used for concerts, lectures, and performances. There's also a cafe on the premises.

● Once through the gates, choose the path that leads south along the eastern edge of Old Yard. You will pass Thayer, University, Weld, and Boylston halls on the left before reaching Wigglesworth Hall, which forms the outer barrier of Harvard. Thayer, Wigglesworth, and Weld (where John F. Kennedy lived as a first-year student) are student residences, while Boylston houses the Department of Romance Languages and Literatures in a modern, completely updated space within the "shell" of the historic Boylston building.

● From Wigglesworth, use the crosswalk to cross Massachusetts Ave. and turn left to walk down Massachusetts. As one of the central arteries of Harvard Square, Mass. Ave. is home to the usual accoutrements of college life: a great bookstore (Harvard Bookstore, at 1256 Massachusetts), a famous burger joint (Mr. & Mrs. Bartley's Burger Cottage, at 1246), and a student place for cheap Chinese food and a crazy drink called a "scorpion bowl" (Hong Kong Restaurant, at 1238). If you're in the mood for something more civilized, try the braised leg of lamb crepe at La Creperie (1154).

As you pass Bow St. on your right, look left across the street at David Phillips's sculpture, *Spiral*, in Quincy Square Park. What used to be bus parking is now a park around a central spiral that leads through the brick into the center of a cut-granite boulder.

● Make a sharp right on Arrow St.

● At Bow St., turn left and then bear right quickly to stay on Bow St.

● Go one block and turn right on Plympton St. to check out Grolier Poetry Book Shop (at 6 Plympton), the country's oldest continually operating bookstore that is devoted entirely to poetry.

● Retrace your steps back to Bow and turn right to continue on Bow. Note the house on the left at 44 Bow St., a wedge-shaped building with a purple and yellow door and a copper roof (the façade looks like a face). This is the Harvard Lampoon Castle, home of the *Harvard Lampoon*, Harvard's literary and humor magazine, where writers like John Updike, Conan O'Brien, and George Plympton honed their satirical skills. Started in 1876 and modeled on the British magazine *Punch*, the *Harvard Lampoon* has a long tradition of parodying both national magazines and the *Harvard Crimson*.

● Where Bow meets Mt. Auburn St., veer right on Mt. Auburn and walk to the Globe Corner Bookstore, at 90 Mt. Auburn. With titles covering everything from the Antilles to Zimbabwe, this travel bookstore is the launch pad for many a great trip.

● Turn right on John F. Kennedy St. to return to Harvard Square. Be sure to duck into Curious George Goes to Wordsworth, at 1 JFK St., a bookstore aimed at your inner child, or perhaps the one with you.

POINTS OF INTEREST

Out of Town News 0 Harvard Square, Cambridge, MA 02138, 617-354-7777

First Unitarian Church of Cambridge 3 Church St., Cambridge, MA 02138, 617-876-7772

Harvard University 1350 Massachusetts Ave, Cambridge, MA 02138, 617-495-1000

Fogg Art Museum 32 Quincy St., Cambridge, MA 02138, 617-495-9400

Harvard Divinity School 14 Divinity Ave., Cambridge, MA 02138, 617-495-5796

Peabody Museum of Archaeology and Ethnology 11 Divinity Ave., Cambridge, MA 02138, 617-496-1027

Harvard Museum of Natural History 26 Oxford St., Cambridge, MA 02138, 617-495-3045

Harvard Bookstore 1256 Massachusetts Ave., Cambridge, MA 02138, 617-661-1515

Mr. & Mrs. Bartley's Burger Cottage 1246 Massachusetts Ave., Cambridge, MA 02138, 617-354-6559

Hong Kong Restaurant 1238 Massachusetts Ave., Cambridge, MA 02138, 617-864-5311

La Creperie 1154 Massachusetts Ave., Cambridge, MA 02138, 617-661-6999

Grolier Poetry Book Shop 6 Plympton St., Cambridge, MA 02138, 617-547-4648

Harvard Lampoon Castle 44 Bow St., Cambridge, MA 02138, 617-495-7801

Globe Corner Bookstore 90 Mt. Auburn Ave., Cambridge, MA 02138, 617-497-6277

Curious George Goes to Wordsworth 1 John F. Kennedy St., Cambridge, MA 02138, 617-498-0062

route summary

1. Begin at Harvard Square and walk north on Massachusetts Ave. to Church St.

2. Cross Massachusetts Ave., enter the campus through the Johnston Gate, and walk straight ahead through the Harvard Yard to University Hall.

3. Cut around the south side of University Hall to the great steps of Widener Library.

4. With your back to the library steps, take the path on the right between Sever and Emerson halls, and continue to Quincy St.

5. Turn left on Quincy St.

6. Turn right on Kirkland St.

7. Make an immediate left on Divinity Ave. and walk to the Peabody Museum of Archaeology and Ethnology.

8. Walk through the museum and connect to the Harvard Museum of Natural History via the third floor, then exit that museum via the front door on Oxford St.

9. Turn left on Oxford St. and, at the corner of Oxford and Kirkland St., take a path into campus and cut south across the campus to Massachusetts Ave.

10. Turn left on Massachusetts Ave.

11. Make a sharp right on Arrow St.

12. Turn left on Bow St.

13. Take a quick jog right up Plympton St. and then retrace your steps to Bow.

14. Turn right to continue on Bow St., then continue on Mt. Auburn St. when Bow merges with Mt. Auburn.

15. Turn right on John F. Kennedy St. to return to Harvard Square.

Harvard Yard

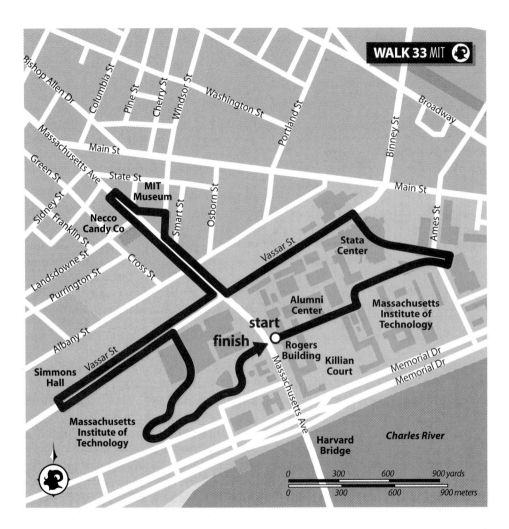

Bishop Allen Dr

Columbia St

Pine St

Cherry St

Windsor St

Washington St

Broadway

Massachusetts Ave

Main St

Portland St

Binney St

Green St

State St

Main St

Ames St

MIT Museum

Smart St

Osborn St

Sidney St

Franklin St

Necco Candy Co

Vassar St

Stata Center

Landsdowne St

Cross St

Purrington St

Alumni Center

Massachusetts Institute of Technology

Albany St

Vassar St

start
finish

Rogers Building

Killian Court

Memorial Dr

Memorial Dr

Simmons Hall

Massachusetts Ave

Massachusetts Institute of Technology

Harvard Bridge

Charles River

0	300	600	900 yards
0	300	600	900 meters

33 MIT: THROUGH THE INFINITE CORRIDOR AND BEYOND

BOUNDARIES: **Massachusetts Ave., Main St., Sidney St., Vassar St., Memorial Dr.**
DISTANCE: **Approx. 2¾ miles**
DIFFICULTY: **Easy**
PARKING: **Paid parking is available at the parking garages at the Marriott Hotel on Broadway and both free and metered street parking can be found on Memorial Dr. and Vassar St.**
PUBLIC TRANSIT: **Central Square or Kendall Square T stations on the Red Line; busses 1, CT1, CT2, and EZ2**

If you associate the Massachusetts Institute of Technology solely with slide rulers and mad scientists, touring the 168-acre Cambridge campus of this premier technical school will enlighten your perspective. Besides its place in history for advances as diverse as gene splicing and the economists' Black-Scholes equation, MIT boasts some of the most renowned modern architecture in Boston. Buildings designed by current "starchitects" like Frank Gehry, as well as masters like I.M. Pei, Alvar Aalto, and Eero Saarinen, dot the campus. You can amble along something called the "Infinite Corridor;" scope sculptures by Pablo Picasso, Alexander Calder, and Henry Moore; and raise a pint in one of the quirkiest (and yet under-the-radar) pubs on the planet.

The best time to go is when classes are in session, and you can feel the energy of thousands of technologically creative minds. And because much of the most interesting parts of this tour are inside, you can save it for late fall or early spring.

● **Begin across the street from the Rogers Building, at 77 Massachusetts Ave., the historic heart of the MIT campus. The inscription over the entranceway, MASSACHUSETTS INSTITUTE OF TECHNOLOGY, FOUNDER WLLIAM BARTON ROGERS, dates from 1916, when MIT relocated from its original home in Boston's Back Bay. The school was founded in 1861 by Rogers, a professor of natural philosophy at the University of Virginia, who wanted to create a place for the study of the "positive sciences." Since then, MIT has been a center for innovation and invention.**

- Enter the massive Rogers Building (which houses numerous departments, classrooms, and offices) by climbing up the wide cement stairs and walking between the Neoclassical columns. Inside, on the left, is a large map of the campus, in case you need to orient yourself.

Once oriented, proceed straight ahead through the Infinite Corridor, which leads through a series of interconnected buildings and provides protection from the frigid Boston winters. Twice a year, light from the setting sun travels the entire, 825-foot length of the hallway, a sometimes spectacular display known as "MIT-henge." (There is, of course, a group and website devoted to analyzing the event and predicting the *exact* time it will occur based on things like the light-bending qualities of the atmosphere and the correct determination of the hallway's azimuth.)

Midway down the corridor, in Building 10, you will come to the Barker Library, which lies beneath the Great Dome in the heart of campus.

- Turn right to go through the doors leading outside to Killian Court, a neat green space bordered by Neoclassical buildings with the names of prominent scientists engraved in a running

Back Story: Playing the Numbers Game

As you catch the whiff of chalk from the equation-etched blackboards, you may notice that pretty much everything is numerically ordered. At this math-centric school, a few buildings carry names, but all are numbered. For example, the Rogers Building is also commonly referred to as "Building 7."

Likewise, MIT departments, which are called "courses" here, use numbers rather than names. Thus, if you ask an MIT senior her major, she might say "Course 5," rather than chemistry, and she will go to most of her classes in Building 18. Department numbers correspond to when the field of study was added to the curriculum—therefore, Course 1 is civil engineering, while Course 24 is linguistics and philosophy.

There is also a system for the order of the building numbers, but it's confusing for anyone without perfect math SAT scores. You'll see the building number on the plates next to most classroom and office doors.

frieze. If the weather's fine, head outside to look across the Charles to Boston. In the far right corner of Killian Court is a bronze Henry Moore statue titled *Three Piece Reclining Figure, Draped*, which was a study for a larger sculpture in New York City's Lincoln Center Plaza.

- Return back inside the Infinite Corridor, and turn right. As you journey down the corridor, you will pass through Building 4.

- At the end of the hallway, enter Building 8 and turn left.

- In Building 8, bear right and walk east through Building 16 into Building 56, which houses the biological engineering and environmental health department. The courtyard to your right, between buildings 56 and 54, was the temporary home of a 1.7-ton Fleming cannon stolen from MIT's West Coast rival, Caltech, in a 2005 hack. The cannon was positioned in the courtyard, facing west—in the exact direction of Caltech. The cannon was eventually returned to Caltech, along with a smaller, toy cannon with a note that read, "This is more your size".

  As you continue through the corridors of Building 56, look for photos of some of the most famous MIT hacks: the various things done to and put on top of the Great Dome, and hacks at the annual Harvard-Yale football game (including a balloon reading "MIT" that rose from the 50-yard line during the 1982 game).

- Continue straight through Building 56, exit the building, and cross the small plaza to enter and walk through Building 66.

Rogers Building at MIT

- At the end of Building 66, leave the indoor comfort of this section of the Infinite Corridor and cross Ames St. to enter Building E15. I.M. Pei, a 1970 MIT graduate, designed the tile-faced building, which houses the MIT Media Lab and List Visual Arts Center. Art at the List tends toward the interactive and cutting edge; exhibits have included such things as "The Fear of Smell—The Smell of Fear," by Norwegian artist Sissel Tolaas. This interactive display had white walls, which, when scratched, gave off odors synthesized from the scents of nine different men who suffer from chronic, acute fear. The gallery is open most days from noon to 6 PM.

- Exit the List Center and walk between buildings 66 and 68 toward the shiny metallic walls of the Ray and Maria Stata Center.

  Opened in 2005, the Gehry-designed Ray and Maria Stata Center (also called buildings 57 and 32) houses the Computer Science and Artificial Intelligence Laboratory, the Laboratory of Information and Decision Systems, and the Department of Linguistics and Philosophy, home of famous linguist and lefty Noam Chomsky, who is now a professor emeritus of MIT.

  Typical of Gehry's high-energy style, there are remarkable views of the building from just about any angle. To truly appreciate this, walk the entire perimeter, which also allows a view of the 350-seat red brick amphitheater along the back. Several lunch trucks frequent the plaza nearby, making this a one-of-a-kind picnic spot on a sunny day.

- Enter the building from the front (along Vassar St.). Inside, sunlight penetrates from multiple angles, and the open design, with exposed staircases and hallway chalkboards scribbled with messages and eureka moments, are meant to foster creativity and collaboration. Walk along the main first-floor corridor to see the series of giant photographs entitled "Earth From Above," by Yann Arthus-Bertrand.

  For another otherworldly experience, take the elevator to the fourth floor and follow the signs to the R&D Pub. Open to the public on Thursday and Friday afternoons and evenings, the R&D Pub is surely one of the coolest (and most secret) watering holes in town. Soft blue lights warm a series of ultra-mod spaces, including two pods hidden away up on a mezzanine level. These pods are smaller, less public spaces

HacKiNG: aN MIT TraDITION

In May of 2004 an MIT campus police car—complete with a flashing blue siren and a blow-up doll of a policewoman at the wheel—mysteriously appeared at the apex of the Great Dome, atop the Alumni Center. There was a half-eaten box of Dunkin' Donuts on the dashboard, a parking ticket on the windshield, and license plate that read "IHTFP"—MIT slang for "I Hate This F****** Place." Later on this tour, you will see the car with the siren still whirling along a wall inside the Stata Center.

"Hacking"—pranks that are clever and ethical (in other words, no person or property is damaged)—have a hallowed place at this school, which is renowned for creativity and know-how. And MIT's Great Dome has been a lightning rod for hacks.

In 1962, students dressed it as the Great Pumpkin (from the *Peanuts* cartoon); in 1996, they made it look like R2-D2; and in 1999, they adorned it with a spinning propeller beanie.

Other buildings have received dark marks from the Harry Potter series, "No Trespassing" signs, or the Batman signal. An important characteristic of hackers is that they are largely anonymous, even after pulling off a successful prank. Officially, the MIT administration frowns on hacking; unofficially, a good hack is one of the most celebrated events on campus. If caught by campus security in the midst of perpetrating a hack, students are counseled to inquire innocently, "Is this the way to Baker House?"

with curving, built-in sofas for conversations on topics more intimate than particle physics and nanotechnology.

Return to the main floor to exit. Before you leave, check out the memorial to Building 20, along the western edge of the building. Building 20 was a temporary facility put on this site during World War II. Although only intended for use during the war and six months after it, Building 20 nonetheless had a distinguished 55-year career as a laboratory for creative geniuses. Radar was invented here.

- Exit the Stata Center via the same doors you used to enter and cross Vassar St. to the Brain and Cognitive Sciences Complex. Completed in 2005, the 411,000-square-foot building, designed by Charles Correa, is the largest neuroscience research center in the world. The building's sun-drenched, five-story atrium is an ethereal spot for lunch or coffee.

- Head west on Vassar.

- Turn right on Massachusetts Ave. and continue two blocks to the MIT Museum, at 265 Massachusetts Ave. The museum has frequently changing exhibits combining science and art. There is also a permanent collection aimed at getting children interested in science.

  From the museum, continue northwest to the yellow brick Novartis Building at 250 Massachusetts Ave. This was the historic factory of New England Confectionary Company, creator of the Necco wafer. If you inhale very deeply, you might just be able to catch a whiff of the peppermint and clove that once perfumed this stretch of Massachusetts Ave.

- Retrace your steps on Massachusetts Ave. to Vassar St. and turn left to walk several blocks to the glistening, geometric Simmons Hall, at 229 Vassar. Designed by architect Steven Holl, the 10-story dorm has a "porous" theme, with large, open blocks throughout the structure. In spite of the fact that the building has received international acclaim and won architectural awards like the Harleston Parker Award from the Boston Society of Architects, students still derisively refer to Simmons as "the chicken coop."

- Retrace your steps on Vassar and turn right on the path in front of the dark red brick Al and Barrie Zesiger Sports and Fitness Center, at 120 Vassar. Enter the center for a glimpse of this great facility, with its Olympic-class pool, massive court areas, and 11,000-square-foot fitness center.

- Exit the Zesiger Center to the south. In front of you, to the left, is the Kresge Auditorium, with its big-tent roof. On the right is a parking lot near the Astroturf soccer fields.

● Walk through the parking lot to Amherst Alley, and follow the alley around to the right (west) to Baker House, a wave-shaped brick dorm on your left. A gem of Modernism completed in 1947, Baker House is one of only two buildings in the United States designed by Finnish architect Alvar Aalto. Most of the building's dorm rooms enjoy sunny exposures and views up and down the Charles. The wooden entrance doors embossed with squares offer a fine example of Aalto's trademark attention to detail.

● From Baker, walk northeast to the center of the green space (known as the Kresge Oval), where there are two examples of work by another modern Finnish architect, Eero Saarinen. Kresge Auditorium, completed in 1955, includes an outer shell, one-eighth of a sphere, which floats free from the rest of building. On the opposite side of the Kresge Oval is the MIT Chapel. Unimpressive from the outside, the chapel radiates a more spiritual feel from the interior, where light appears in twinkling dots along the round walls.

● From the chapel, head north toward the Stratton Student Center (where you can refuel at student favorite Anna's Taqueria), or turn right on the pathway just before the center to return to the starting point across the street from the Rogers Building.

POINTS OF Interest

Massachusetts Institute of Technology 77 Massachusetts Ave., Cambridge, MA 02139, 617-253-4795

List Visual Arts Center 20 Ames St., Cambridge, MA 02139, 617-253-4680

R&D Pub, Ray and Maria Stata Center 32 Vassar St., Cambridge, MA 02139, 617-253-5073

MIT Museum 265 Massachusetts Ave., Cambridge, MA 02139, 617-253-4444

Anna's Taqueria Building W20, 77 Massachusetts Ave., Cambridge, MA 02139, 617-324-2662

route summary

1. Enter the Rogers Building at 77 Massachusetts Ave., and follow the Infinite Corridor through buildings 7, 10, 4, 8, 16, and 56.

2. Exit Building 56, cross the small plaza to enter Building 66, and continue through Building 66.

3. Exit Building 66 and cross Ames St. to enter Building E15 (the List Visual Arts Center).

4. Exit Building E15 and walk between buildings 66 and 68 to enter the Ray and Maria Stata Center.

5. Exit the Stata Center at Vassar St. and head west on Vassar.

6. Turn right on Massachusetts Ave. and walk to the MIT Museum at 256 Massachusetts Ave. and then the Novartis Building at 250 Massachusetts..

7. Retrace your steps on Massachusetts and turn right on Vassar St.

8. Walk to 229 Vassar, and then retrace your steps on Vassar to the Al and Barrie Zesiger Sports and Fitness Center, at 120 Vassar.

9. Turn right on the path in front of the Zesiger Center and walk through the center to exit on its south side.

10. Walk through the parking lot on your right to Amherst Alley, and follow the alley as it bends right (west) to Baker House.

11. From Baker, walk northeast on the pathway, past the Kresge Auditorium and the MIT Chapel, toward the Stratton Student Center.

12. Turn right on the pathway just before the student center to return to your starting point at the Rogers Building.

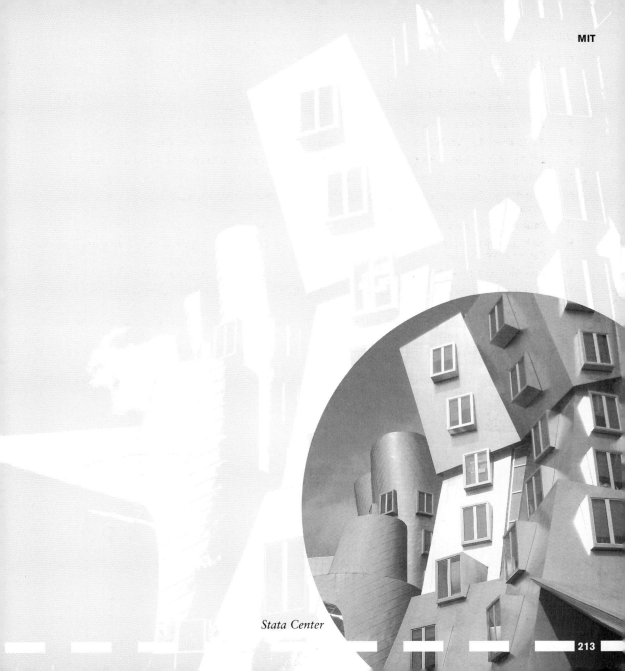

Stata Center

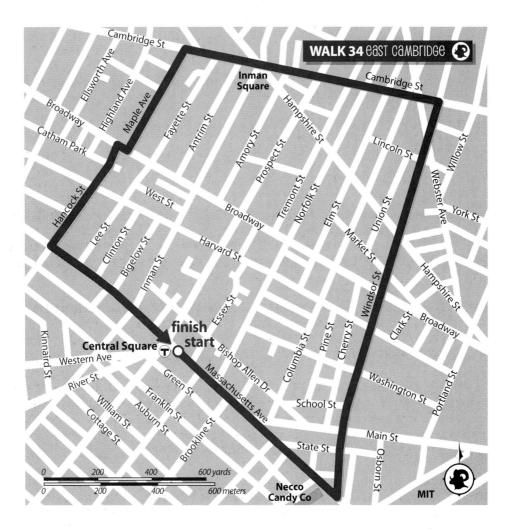

WALK 34 east cambridge

Cambridge St

Inman Square

Cambridge St

Ellsworth Ave

Highland Ave

Maple Ave

Fayette St

Antrim St

Hampshire St

Lincoln St

Willow St

Broadway

Catham Park

Amory St

Prospect St

Tremont St

Norfolk St

Elm St

Market St

Union St

Webster Ave

York St

Hancock St

West St

Broadway

Windsor St

Hampshire St

Lee St

Clinton St

Bigelow St

Harvard St

Clark St

Broadway

Inman St

Essex St

**finish
start**

Central Square Ⓣ ○

Kinnaird St

Western Ave

Green St

Bishop Allen Dr

Columbia St

Pine St

Cherry St

River St

Franklin St

Massachusetts Ave

Washington St

Portland St

William St

Auburn St

Brookline St

School St

Main St

Cottage St

State St

Osborn St

0   200   400   600 yards

0   200   400   600 meters

**Necco
Candy Co**

MIT

34 east cambridge: Bands, Beers, and Ben franklin in red sneakers

BOUNDARIES: Massachusetts Ave., Windsor St., Cambridge St., Hancock St.
DISTANCE: Approx 2¾ miles
DIFFICULTY: Easy
PARKING: There is a paid parking lot at 438 Green St.
PUBLIC TRANSIT: Central Square T Station on the Red Line; busses 1, CT1, and 64

Harvard Square may be home to the literati and cultural elite, but move farther east, and Cambridge is a vibrant mix of people, ethnic restaurants, funky music clubs, and hipster bars. Save this walk for those first few warm evenings in spring, when the collective masses begin to hum with the excitement and anticipation of the coming summer. The best plan is to do the entire walk in the late afternoon, scoping out the venues with the best acts for the night, and then have dinner at one of the myriad excellent choices, finishing just in time to return to the bar of your choice before the opening act plugs in their amps.

● Start inside the Central Square T Station and note the tile murals by Elizabeth Mapelli on the walls of the station. The fused-glass murals abstractly represent several ethnic groups that have made their homes in Central Square—East Indian, Mediterranean, African, Japanese, Chinese, Irish, English, Scottish, and Polish.

Once aboveground, head east on Massachusetts Ave. If you need a little something before you start on this circumnavigation of East Cambridge, stop by the Central Kitchen, at 567 Massachusetts, or the Phoenix Landing, at 512. Central Kitchen offers upscale goodies like braised lamb shanks at reasonable prices, while Phoenix Landing updates the traditional Irish pub.

As you pass the Middle East, at 472, check out the listing for what's playing later on its three stages. There's a big one downstairs for large acts, while upstairs are two more intimate venues. You can also check out T.T. the Bear's Place, at 10 Brookline St. (just past the wild mural on the left), by turning right on Brookline

St. T.T. the Bear's doesn't look like much from the outside, but it's popular for seeing local and national acts.

The final bar to check out along Massachusetts Ave. is the Miracle of Science Bar and Grill, at 321 Massachusetts Ave. True to its name, this watering hole is filled with cool science tricks and the fascinating people who understand them. Just try ordering off a menu that's designed as a periodic table.

● Turn left on Windsor St. for the hike up to Cambridge St. It's a bit of a haul, but this quiet, leafy street is a peaceful diversion. If you get wiped out, stop in to the B-Side Lounge (92 Hampshire, on the corner of Windsor), with its cool, retro rockabilly jukebox.

● Turn left on Cambridge St. and continue to the hustle and bustle of Inman Square, where Cambridge, Inman, and Hampshire streets all intersect in a colorful medley of ethnic cuisine—Thai, Mexican, Irish, and Indian. If you need just a small snack, duck around the corner to Rosie's Bakery, at 243 Hampshire St. This sweet spot serves cheerfully decorated cakes and cookies, brownies, and bars. You can take your treat across Hampshire St. to the little park on the corner of Hampshire and Cambridge.

From Rosie's, cross Cambridge carefully at the sidewalk. On the west-facing wall of the Inman Square Firehouse, note the mural of Benjamin Franklin (in the red sneakers) and George Washington (holding the pails) in among the members of the 1976 Engine #5 company.

Continue west on Cambridge.

● Turn left on Maple Ave.

● At Broadway, make a short jog to the right, followed by a quick left on Hancock St. Follow Hancock all the way down to Massachusetts Ave., where you'll find the green and maroon Plough & Stars. This is a real Irish bar, so duck into the darkness, pull up a stool, and order your Guinness. If you're lucky, there'll be a weekend soccer match on the TV.

● Turn left on Massachusetts Ave. About a block down, on the right, is a popular place to mix your philosophy and your beer: the People's Republik, at 876 Massachusetts. Don't let the brightly painted exterior fool you; inside it is dark and informal—perfect for planning a revolution.

As you continue down Massachusetts Ave., you will pass the Cambridge City Hall (on the left, at 795) and the Cambridge Post Office (on the right, at 770). These two buildings used to form the heart of Cambridge, before commercialism pulled it down to Central Square.

● Before you end the tour at Central Square, take a moment to check out the brass and frosted glass towers inscribed with the hopes and dreams of various Cantabrigians. This Central Square art installation was created in 1995 by Ritsuko Taho, who spent five months collecting the "dream statements." The cylinders glow from within at night.

POINTS OF INTEREST

Central Kitchen 567 Massachusetts Ave., Cambridge, MA 02139, 617-491-5599

Phoenix Landing 512 Massachusetts Ave., Cambridge, MA 02139, 617-576-6260

Middle East 472 Massachusetts Ave., Cambridge, MA 02139, 617-492-9181

T.T. the Bear's Place 10 Brookline St., Cambridge, MA 02139, 617-492-2327

Miracle of Science Bar and Grill 321 Massachusetts Ave., Cambridge, MA 02139, 617-868-2866

B-Side Lounge 92 Hampshire St., Cambridge, MA 02139, 617-354-0766

Rosie's Bakery 243 Hampshire St., Cambridge, MA 02139, 617-491-9488

Plough & Stars 912 Massachusetts Ave., Cambridge, MA 02139, 617-576-0032

People's Republik 876 Massachusetts Ave., Cambridge, MA 02139, 617-491-6969

route summary

1. Begin at the Central Square T station and head east on Massachusetts Ave.
2. Turn left on Windsor St.
3. Turn left on Cambridge St.
4. Turn left on Maple Ave.
5. Turn right on Broadway.
6. Make an immediate left on Hancock St.
7. Turn left on Massachusetts Ave. to return to the Central Square T Station.

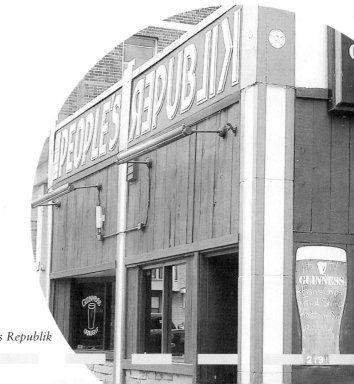

People's Republik

Appendix 1: WALKS BY THEME

GReeN SPaceS

Rose Fitzgerald Kennedy Greenway
and the Waterfront (Walk 6)
Public Garden and Boston Common
(Walk 9)
Commonwealth Avenue (Walk 10)
Brook Farm (Walk 17)
Roslindale and the Arnold Arboretum
(Walk 18)
Jamaica Plain (Walk 19)
Back Bay Fens (Walk 22)
Charles River Basin (Walk 24)
Belle Isle Marsh and Suffolk Downs
(Walk 27)
Spectacle Island (Walk 28)
Charles River Reservation (Walk 29)
Fresh Pond (Walk 30)
North Cambridge (Walk 31)

BLue SPaceS

Rose Fitzgerald Kennedy Greenway
and the Waterfront (Walk 6)
South Boston (Walk 14)
Castle Island (Walk 15)
Columbia Point (Walk 16)
Charles River Basin (Walk 24)

East Boston (Walk 26)
Belle Isle Marsh and Suffolk Downs
(Walk 27)
Spectacle Island (Walk 28)
Charles River Reservation (Walk 29)
Fresh Pond (Walk 30)

HISTORIC areas

Beacon Hill (Walk 1)
North End (Walk 2)
Haymarket, Faneuil Hall Marketplace,
and Government Center (Walk 3)
Financial District (Walk 4)
Downtown (Walk 5)
Chinatown (Walk 7)
Bay Village (Walk 8)
Public Garden and Boston Common
(Walk 9)
Commonwealth Avenue (Walk 10)
Back Bay (Walk 11)
Copley Square (Walk 12)
South End (Walk 13)
Castle Island (Walk 15)
Columbia Point (Walk 16)
Brook Farm (Walk 17)
Roslindale and the Arnold Arboretum
(Walk 18)
Fenway Park (Walk 23)
Charlestown (Walk 25)

DINING, SHOPPING, AND ENTERTAINMENT

Beacon Hill (Walk 1)
North End (Walk 2)
Haymarket, Faneuil Hall Marketplace, and Government Center (Walk 3)
Financial District (Walk 4)
Downtown (Walk 5)
Chinatown (Walk 7)
Back Bay (Walk 11)
Copley Square (Walk 12)
South End (Walk 13)
East Cambridge (Walk 34)

AROUND CAMPUS

Boston College and Chestnut Hill (Walk 21)
North Cambridge (Walk 31)
Harvard Square and University (Walk 32)
MIT (Walk 33)

AROUND TOWN

Beacon Hill (Walk 1)
North End (Walk 2)
Haymarket, Faneuil Hall Marketplace, and Government Center (Walk 3)
Financial District (Walk 4)
Downtown (Walk 5)
Chinatown (Walk 7)
Bay Village (Walk 8)
Back Bay (Walk 11)
Jamaica Plain (Walk 19)
Newton Centre (Walk 20)
North Cambridge (Walk 31)

Appendix 2: POINTS OF INTEREST

FOOD AND DRINK

Anna's Taqueria Building W20, 77 Massachusetts Ave., Cambridge, MA 02139, 617-324-2662 (Walk 33)

Anthony's Pier 4 140 Northern Ave., Boston, MA 02210, 617-482-6262 (Walk 14)

Antico Forno 93 Salem St., Boston, MA 02113, 617-723-6733 (Walk 2)

B & G Oysters 550 Tremont St., Boston, MA 02118, 617-423-0550 (Walk 13)

B-Side Lounge 92 Hampshire St., Cambridge, MA 02139, 617-354-0766 (Walk 34)

Barking Crab Restaurant 88 Sleeper St., Boston, MA 02210, 617-426-2722 (Walk 14)

Bella's Market 75 Maverick Square, East Boston, MA 02128, 617-567-7152 (Walk 25)

Boston Beer Works 61 Brookline Ave., Boston, MA 02215, 617-536-2337 (Walk 23)

Boston Halal Meat Market 114 Blackstone St., Boston, MA 02109, 617-367-6181 (Walk 3)

Bova Bakery 134 Salem St., Boston, MA 02113, 617-523-5601 (Walk 2)

Brown Sugar Cafe 129 Jersey St., Boston, MA 02215, 617-266-2928 (Walk 23)

Butcher Shop 552 Tremont St., Boston, MA 02118, 617-423-4800 (Walk 13)

Cafe Amsterdam 517 Columbus Ave., Boston, MA 02118, 617-437-6400 (Walk 13)

Cafe Bella Vita 30 Charles St., Boston, MA 02114, 617-720-4505 (Walk 1)

Cask'n Flagon 62 Brookline Ave., Boston, MA 02215, 617-536-4840 (Walk 23)

Central Kitchen 567 Massachusetts Ave., Cambridge, MA 02139, 617-491-5599 (Walk 34)

Columbus Cafe and Bar 535 Columbus Ave., Boston, MA 02118, 617-247-9001 (Walk 13)

Dairy Fresh Candies 57 Salem St., Boston, MA 02113, 617-742-2639 (Walk 2)

DeLuca's Market 11 Charles St., Boston, MA 02114, 617-227-2117 (Walk 1)

Durgin-Park North Market, Boston, MA 02109, 617-227-2038 (Walk 3)

Eldo Cake House Bakery 36 Harrison Ave., Boston, MA 02111, 617-350-7977 (Walk 7)

Emack & Bolio's 290 Newbury St., Boston, MA 02115, 617-536-7127 (Walk 11)

Finale 1 Columbus Ave., Boston, MA 02116, 617-423-3184 (Walk 8)

Fornax Bread Company Incorporated 27 Corinth St., Roslindale, MA 02131, 617-325-8852 (Walk 18)

Haley House Corner Shop 23 Dartmouth St., Boston, MA 02118, 617-236-8132 (Walk 13)

Hamersley's Bistro 553 Tremont St., Boston, MA 02118, 617-423-2700 (Walk 13)

Haymarket Farmer's Market Corner of Blackstone and Hanover streets, Boston, MA 02109 (Walk 3)

Hin Shing Bakery 67 Beach St., Boston, MA 02111, 617-451-1162 (Walk 7)

Hi-Rise Bakery 208 Concord Ave., Cambridge, MA 02138, 617-876-8766 (Walk 31)

Hong Kong Eatery 79 Harrison Ave., Boston, MA 02111, 617-423-0838 (Walk 7)

Hong Kong Restaurant 1238 Massachusetts Ave., Cambridge, MA 02138, 617-864-5311 (Walk 32)

House of Siam 542 Columbus Ave., Boston, MA 02118, 617-267-1755 (Walk 13)

J.P. Licks 659 Centre St., Jamaica Plain, MA 02130, 617-524-6740 (Walk 19)

James Hook and Company 15–17 Northern Ave., Boston, MA 02210, 617-423-5500 (Walk 6)

Johnny's Luncheonette 30 Langley Rd., Newton, MA 02459, 617-527-3223 (Walk 20)

La Creperie 1154 Massachusetts Ave., Cambridge, MA 02138, 617-661-6999 (Walk 32)

La Sultana 40 Maverick Square, East Boston, MA 02128, 617-568-9999 (Walk 26)

Lizzy's Ice Cream 29 Church St., Cambridge, MA 02138, 617-354-2911 (Walk 29)

L'Osteria 104 Salem St., Boston, MA 02113, 617-723-7847 (Walk 2)

Lucky House Seafood Restaurant 10 Tyler St., Boston, MA 02111, 617-338-9038 (Walk 7)

Marco Polo 274 Summer St., Boston, MA 02210, 617-695-9039 (Walk 14)

Middle East 472 Massachusetts Ave., Cambridge, MA 02139, 617-492-9181 (Walk 34)

Mike's Pastry 300 Hanover St., Boston, MA 02113, 617-742-3050 (Walk 2)

Milk Street Cafe Post Office Square at the intersection of Franklin and Congress Sts., Boston, MA 02109, 617-542-3663 (Walk 4)

Miracle of Science Bar and Grill 321 Massachusetts Ave., Cambridge, MA 02139, 617-868-2866 (Walk 34)

Mr. & Mrs. Bartley's Burger Cottage 1246 Massachusetts Ave., Cambridge, MA 02138, 617-354-6559 (Walk 32)

Olives 10 City Square, Charlestown, MA 02129, 617-242-1999 (Walk 25)

Other Side Cosmic Cafe 407 Newbury St., Boston, MA 02115, 617-536-9477 (Walk 11)

Parish Cafe 361 Boylston St., Boston, MA 02116, 617-247-4777 (Walk 11)

Peach Farm 4 Tyler St., Boston, MA 02111, 617-482-3332 (Walk 7)

Peet's Coffee and Tea 776 Beacon St., Newton, MA 02459, 617-244-1577 (Walk 20)

People's Republik 876 Massachusetts Ave., Cambridge, MA 02139, 617-491-6969 (Walk 34)

Pho Pasteur 682 Washington St., Boston, MA 02111, 617-482-7467 (Walk 7)

Phoenix Landing 512 Massachusetts Ave., Cambridge, MA 02139, 617-576-6260 (Walk 34)

Plough & Stars 912 Massachusetts Ave., Cambridge, MA 02139, 617-576-0032 (Walk 34)

R&D Pub, Ray and Maria Stata Center 32 Vassar St., Cambridge, MA 02139, 617-253-5073 (Walk 33)

Rachel's Kitchen 12 Church St., Boston, MA 02116, 617-423-3447 (Walk 8)

Rosie's Bakery 243 Hampshire St., Cambridge, MA 02139, 617-491-9488 (Walk 34)

Sibling Rivalry 525 Tremont St., Boston, MA 02118, 617-338-5338 (Walk 13)

Smith & Wollensky 101 Arlington St., Boston, MA 02116, 617-423-1112 (Walk 8)

Solera 12 Corinth St., Roslindale, MA 02131, 617-469-4005 (Walk 18)

Sophia's Grotto Cafe 22 Birch St., Roslindale, MA 02131, 617-323-4595 (Walk 18)

South End Buttery 314 Shawmut Ave., Boston, MA 02118, 617-482-1015 (Walk 13)

Sullivan's Restaurant 2000 William J. Day Blvd., South Boston, MA 02127, 617-268-5685 (Walk 15)

Taqueria Cancun 192 Sumner St., East Boston, MA 02128, 617-567-4449 (Walk 26)

T.T. the Bear's Place 10 Brookline St., Cambridge, MA 02139, 617-492-2327 (Walk 34)

Union Oyster House 41 Union St., Boston, MA 02108, 617-227-2750 (Walk 3)

Village Market 30 Corinth St., Roslindale, MA 02131, 617-327-2588 (Walk 18)

Warren Tavern 2 Pleasant St., Charlestown, MA 02129, 617-241-8142 (Walk 25)

West Street Grille 15 West St., Boston, MA 02110, 617-423-0300 (Walk 5)

Wonder Spice Cafe 697 Centre St., Jamaica Plain, MA 02130, 617-522-020 (Walk 19)

HOTELS

Boston Harbor Hotel 70 Rowes Wharf, Boston, MA 02110, 617-439-7000 (Walk 6)

Boston Marriott Hotel 296 State St., Boston, MA 02109, 617-227-0800 (Walk 6)

Four Seasons Hotel 200 Boylston St., Boston, MA 02116, 617-338-4400 (Walk 9)

Intercontinental Hotel 510 Atlantic Ave., Boston, MA 02210, 617-747-1000 (Walk 14)

Langham Hotel 250 Franklin St., Boston, MA 02109, 617-451-1900 (Walk 4)

Omni Parker House Hotel 60 School St., Boston, MA 02108, 617-227-8600 (Walk 5)

ENTERTAINMENT AND NIGHTLIFE

American Repertory Theatre 64 Brattle St., Cambridge, MA 02138, 617-547-8300 (Walk 32)

Fenway Park 4 Yawkey Way, Boston, MA 02215, 877-733-7699 (Walk 23)

Harvard Stadium 95 N. Harvard St., Allston, MA 02134, 617-495-1000 (Walk 29)

Publick Theatre 1175A Soldiers Field Rd., Brighton, MA 02135, 617-782-5425 (Walk 29)

Suffolk Downs 111 Waldemar Ave., East Boston, MA 02128, 617-567-3900 (Walk 27)

TD Banknorth Garden 100 Legends Way., Boston, MA 02114, 617-624-1050 (Walk 2)

MUSEUMS AND GALLERIES

Boston Tea Party Ships and Museum Congress St. Bridge, Boston, MA 02210. This is closed for renovation until summer 2009. (Walk 14)

Children's Museum 300 Congress St., Boston, MA 02210, 617-426-8855 (Walk 14)

Commonwealth Museum 220 Morrissey Blvd., Boston, MA 02125, 617-727-9268 (Walk 16)

Fogg Art Museum 32 Quincy St., Cambridge, MA 02138, 617-495-9400 (Walk 32)

Gibson House Museum 137 Beacon St., Boston, MA 02116, 617-267-6338 (Walk 10)

Harvard Museum of Natural History 26 Oxford St., Cambridge, MA 02138, 617-495-3045 (Walk 32)

Institute of Contemporary Art 100 Northern Ave., Boston, MA 02210, 617-478-3101 (Walk 14)

Isabella Stewart Gardner Museum 280 Fenway, Boston, MA 02115, 617-566-1401 (Walk 22)

List Visual Arts Center 20 Ames St., Cambridge, MA 02139, 617 253-4680 (Walk 33)

Massachusetts Archives 220 Morrissey Blvd., Boston, MA 02125, 617-727-2816 (Walk 16)

MIT Museum 265 Massachusetts Ave., Cambridge, MA 02139, 617-253-4444 (Walk 33)

Museum of African American History 46 Joy St., Boston, MA 02114, 617-725-0022 (Walk 1)

Museum of Fine Arts 465 Huntington Ave., Boston, MA 02115, 617-267-9300 (Walk 22)

Museum of Science 1 Science Park, Boston, MA 02114, 617-723-2500 (Walk 24)

New England Aquarium Central Wharf, Boston, MA 02110, 617-973-5200 (Walk 6)

Nichols House Museum 55 Mt. Vernon St., Boston, MA 02114, 617-227-6993 (Walk 1)

Peabody Museum of Archaeology and Ethnology 11 Divinity Ave., Cambridge, MA 02138, 617-496-1027 (Walk 32)

educational and cultural centers

Appalachian Mountain Club 5 Joy St., Boston, MA 02114, 617-523-0636 (Walk 1)

Boston Athenaeum 10½ Beacon St., Boston, MA 02108, 617-227-0270 (Walk 5)

Boston Center for the Arts 539 Tremont St., Boston, MA 02118, 617-426-5000 (Walk 13)

Boston College 140 Commonwealth Ave., Chestnut Hill, MA 02467, 617-552-3100 (Walk 21)

Boston Duck Tours 3 Copley Pl. (main office), Boston, MA 02116, 617-267-DUCK (Walk 24)

Boston Globe **headquarters** 135 Morrissey Blvd., Boston, MA 02125, 617-929-2000 (Walk 16)

Boston Public Central Library 700 Boylston St., Boston, MA 02116, 617-536-5400 (Walk 11)

Cambridge Public Library 245 Concord Ave., Cambridge, MA 02138, 617-349-4017 (Walk 31)

Charles Street Meeting House 70 Charles St., Boston, MA 02114 (Walk 1)

Community Boating 21 David Mugar Way, Boston, MA 02114, 617-523-1038 (Walk 24)

Courageous Sailing Center Jamaica Pond Boathouse, Jamaica Plain, MA 02130, 617-522-5061 (Walk 19)

Eliot School of Fine and Applied Arts 24 Eliot St., Jamaica Plain, MA 02130, 617-524-3313 (Walk 19)

Footlight Club 7A Eliot St., Jamaica Plain, MA 02130, 617-524-6506 (Walk 19)

Fort Point Arts Connect Gallery 300 Summer St., Boston, MA 02210, 617-423-4299 (Walk 14)

French Library and Cultural Center 53 Marlborough St., Boston, MA 02116, 617-912-0400 (Walk 10)

Harvard Divinity School 14 Divinity Ave., Cambridge, MA 02138, 617-495-5796 (Walk 32)

Harvard Lampoon Castle 44 Bow St., Cambridge, MA 02138, 617-495-7801 (Walk 32)

Harvard University Massachusetts Ave, Cambridge, MA 02138, 617-495-1000 (Walk 32)

Hatch Memorial Shell On the Esplanade, Boston, MA 02114, 617-727-1300 (Walk 24)

John F. Kennedy Presidential Library and Museum Columbia Point, Boston, MA 02125, 617-514-1600 (Walk 16)

Mary Baker Eddy Library 200 Massachusetts Ave., Boston, MA 02115, 888-222-3711 (Walk 12)

Massachusetts Institute of Technology 77 Massachusetts Ave., Cambridge, MA 02139, 617-253-4795 (Walk 33)

New England Historic Genealogical Society 101 Newbury St., Boston, MA 02116, 617-536-5740 (Walk 11)

Piers Park Sailing Center 95 Marginal Rd., East Boston, MA 02128, 617-561-6677 (Walk 26)

UMass Boston 100 Morrissey Blvd., Boston, MA 02125, 617-287-5000 (Walk 16)

HISTORIC LANDMARKS AND MONUMENTS

Boston National Historical Park Charlestown Navy Yard, Charlestown, MA 02129, 617-242-5601 (Walk 25)

Brook Farm National Historic Site 670 Baker St., West Roxbury, MA 02132, 617-698-1802 (Walk 17)

Bunker Hill Monument Monument Square, Charlestown, MA 02129, 617-242-5641 (Walk 25)

Bunker Hill Pavilion 55 Constitution Rd., Charlestown, MA 02129, 617-242-5601 (Walk 25)

Copp's Hill Burying Ground Corner of Snowhill and Hull streets, Boston, MA 02113, 617-635-4505 (Walk 2)

Fort Independence William J. Day Blvd., South Boston, MA 02127, 617-268-8870 (Walk 15)

Longfellow House 105 Brattle St., Cambridge, MA 02138, 617-876-4491 (Walk 29)

Massachusetts State House 1 Beacon St., Boston, MA 02133, 617-727-3676 (Walk 5)

National Historical Park visitors center 15 State St., Boston, MA 02109, 617-242-5642 (Walk 4)

Old Corner Bookstore Building 3 School St., Boston, MA 02108 (Walk 5)

Old South Meeting House 310 Washington St., Boston, MA 02108, 617-482-6439 (Walk 5)

Old State House 206 Washington St., Boston, MA 02109, 617-720-1713 (Walk 4)

Paul Revere House Museum/Pierce-Hichborn House 19 North Square, Boston, MA 02113, 617-523-2338 (Walk 2)

USS *Cassin Young* Charlestown Navy Yard, Charlestown, MA 02129, 617-242-5644 (Walk 25)

USS *Constitution* Charlestown Navy Yard, Charlestown, MA 02129, 617-242-7511 (Walk 25)

SPIRITUAL INSTITUTIONS

Arlington Street Church 351 Boylston St., Boston, MA 02116, 617-536-7050 (Walk 11)
Concord Baptist Church 190 Warren Ave., Boston, MA 02118, 617-266-8062 (Walk 13)
Emmanuel Church 15 Newbury St., Boston, MA 02116, 617-536-3355 (Walk 11)
First and Second Church of Boston 66 Marlborough St., Boston, MA 02116, 617-267-6730 (Walk 10)
First Unitarian Church of Cambridge 3 Church St., Cambridge, MA 02138, 617-876-7772 (Walk 32)
King's Chapel 58 Tremont St., Boston, MA 02108, 617-523-1749 (Walk 5)
Old North Church 193 Salem St., Boston, MA 02113, 617-523-6676 (Walk 2)
Park Street Church 1 Park St., Boston, MA 02108, 617-523-3383 (Walk 5)
St. Stephen's Church 401 Hanover St., Boston, MA 02113, 617-523-1230 (Walk 2)
Vilna Shul/Boston Center for Jewish Heritage 18 Phillips St., Boston, MA 02114, 617-523-2324 (Walk 1)

SHOPPING

Adams Fireplace Shop 505 Concord Ave., Cambridge, MA 02138, 617-547-3100 (Walk 31)
Best Cellars 745 Boylston St., Boston, MA 02116, 617-266-2900 (Walk 11)
Boing! 729 Centre St., Jamaica Plain, MA 02130, 617-522-7800 (Walk 19)
Boston Stone Souvenir Shop 9 Marshall St., Boston, MA 02108, 617-227-6968 (Walk 3)
Brattle Books 9 West St., Boston, MA 02110, 617-542-0210 (Walk 5)
Bryn Mawr Bookstore 373 Huron Ave., Cambridge, MA 02138, 617-661-1770 (Walk 31)
Cambridgeside Galleria Mall 100 Cambridgeside Pl., Cambridge, MA 02141, 617-621-8666 (Walk 24)
Copley Place 2 Copley Pl. Boston, MA 02116, 617-369-5000 (Walk 12)
Copley Square Farmer's Market Copley Square along St. James Ave., Boston, MA 02116,
    Tuesdays and Fridays, 11 AM to 6 PM (Walk 12)
Crate and Barrel 777 Boylston St., Boston, MA 02116, 617-262-8700 (Walk 11)
Curious George Goes to Wordsworth 1 John F. Kennedy St., Cambridge, MA 02138, 617-498-0062
    (Walk 32)
Emack & Bolio's 290 Newbury St., Boston, MA 02115, 617-247-8772 (Walk 11)
Faneuil Hall Marketplace Clinton St. and North St., Boston, MA 02109, 617-523-1300 (Walk 3)
Fishmonger 252 Huron Ave., Cambridge, MA 02138, 617-661-4834 (Walk 31)
Globe Corner Bookstore 90 Mt. Auburn Ave., Cambridge, MA 02138, 617-497-6277 (Walk 32)
Grolier Poetry Book Shop 6 Plympton St., Cambridge, MA 02138, 617-547-4648 (Walk 32)

Harvard Bookstore 1256 Massachusetts Ave., Cambridge, MA 02138, 617-661-1515 (Walk 32)
Henry Bear's Park 361 Huron Ave., Cambridge, MA 02138, 617-547-8424 (Walk 31)
John Hancock Tower 200 Clarendon St., Boston, MA 02116, 617-572-6429 (Walk 12)
Life is Good 283 Newbury St., Boston, MA 02116, 617-867-8900 (Walk 11)
Louis Boston 234 Berkeley St., Boston, MA 02116, 800-225-5135 (Walk 11)
Newbury Comics 332 Newbury St., Boston, MA 02115, 617-236-4930 (Walk 11)
Niketown 200 Newbury St., Boston, MA 02116, 617-267-3400 (Walk 11)
Out of Town News 0 Harvard Square, Cambridge, MA 02138, 617-354-7777 (Walk 32)
Party Shop Incorporated 42 Langley Rd., Newton, MA 02459, 617-244-8382 (Walk 20)
Prudential Center 800 Boylston St., Boston, MA 02199, 617-236-3100 (Walk 12)
Restoration Hardware 711 Boylston St., Boston, MA 02116, 617-578-0088 (Walk 11)
Souvenir Shop 19 Yawkey Way, Boston, MA 02215, 617-426-8686 (Walk 23)
Trident Booksellers and Cafe 338 Newbury St., Boston, MA 02115, 617-267-8688 (Walk 11)

Parks and Gardens

Arnold Arboretum Hunnewell visitors center 125 Arborway, Jamaica Plain, MA 02130, 617-524-1718 (Walk 18)
Back Bay Fens Between Fenway and Park Dr., Boston, MA 02115 (Walk 22)
Bay Village Park Corner of Fayette St. and Broadway, Boston, MA 02116 (Walk 8)
Belle Isle Marsh Reservation Bennington St. (across from Suffolk Downs), East Boston, MA 02128, 617-727-5350 (Walk 27)
Boston Common visitors center 147 Tremont St., Boston, MA 02108, 617-536-4100 (Walk 9)
Boston Harbor Islands National Recreation Area 617-223-8666 (Walk 28)
Brewer St. Tot Lot Brewer St., between Burroughs St. and Thomas St., Jamaica Plain, MA 02130 (Walk 19)
Chestnut Hill Reservation Chestnut Hill Dr. and Beacon St., Allston/Brighton, MA 02134, 617-333-7404 (Walk 21)
Chinatown Park Corner of Essex St. and Surface Rd., Boston, MA 02111 (Walk 7)
Christopher Columbus Park Corner of Cross St. and Atlantic Ave., Boston, MA 02109, 617-635-4505 (Walk 6)
Fenway Victory Gardens Corner of Boylston St. and Park Dr., Boston, MA 02115, 617-267-6650 (Walk 22)
Frog Pond Boston Common, Boston, MA 02108, 617-635-2120 (Walk 9)
Harriet Tubman Park Columbus Ave. and Warren St., Boston, MA 02118, 617-266-0022 (Walk 13)

Jamaica Pond Nature Center Jamaica Pond Boathouse, Jamaica Plain, MA 02130, 617-522-5061 (Walk 19)

John F. Kennedy Park Memorial Dr., Cambridge, MA 02167, 617-727-5250 (Walk 29)

Kingsley Park Fresh Pond Pkwy., Cambridge, MA 02138, 617-349-4793 (Walk 30)

Langone Recreational Complex Commercial St. at Charter St., Boston, MA 02113, 617-626-1250 (Walk 2)

Mayor Thomas W. Danehy Park 99 Sherman St., Cambridge, MA 02138, 617-349-4895 (Walk 31)

Rose Fitzgerald Kennedy Greenway Along Atlantic Ave. between Summer and State streets, Boston, MA 02109, 617-292-0020 (Walk 6)

Swan Boats Public Garden Lagoon, Boston, MA 02108, 617-522-1966 (Walk 9)

MISCELLANEOUS

Boston Convention and Exhibition Center 415 Summer St., Boston, MA 02210, 617-954-2000 (Walk 14)

Boston School of Modern Languages 814 South St., Roslindale, MA 02131, 617-325-2760 (Walk 18)

Independence Wharf 470 Atlantic Ave., Boston, MA 02210, 617-273-8000 (Walk 14)

Moakley Federal Courthouse 1 Courthouse Way, Boston, MA 02210, 617-261-2440 (Walk 14)

South Station T Station 245 Summer St., Boston, MA 02110, 617-222-5215 (Walk 6)

Walter J. Sullivan Water Purification Facility 250 Fresh Pond Pkwy., Cambridge, MA 02138, 617-349-6489 (Walk 30)

World Trade Center Boston 200 Seaport Blvd., Boston, MA 02210, 617-385-5000 (Walk 14)

INDEX

(*Italicized* page numbers indicate photos.)

aBOUT THE auTHOr

Robert Todd Felton recently took a short break from a decade of teaching English to give freelance writing a try. Four years and three books later, it seems increasingly unlikely that he will go back to teaching. He is having too much fun writing about the transcendentalists of New England (his first book), Irish literature (his second book), and now, walking around the great city of beans and baseball champs, Boston. Todd has also penned stories on hiking with Kerouac, the hidden beer gardens of Salzburg, and how to plan that great backpacking trip. When not finding excuses to go places and do things, Todd can be found in front of his computer at home in Amherst, Massachusetts, where he lives with his wife and two boys.

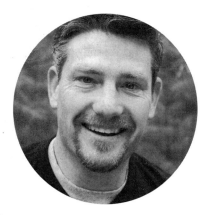